Early Intervention in Psychiatric Disorders Across Cultures

Early Intervention in Psychiatric Disorders Across Cultures

Edited by

Eric Y.H. Chen

Head and Professor, Department of Psychiatry, University of Hong Kong, Queen Mary Hospital, Hong Kong, China

Antonio Ventriglio

Psychiatrist, Department of Mental Health, Department of Clinical and Experimental Medicine, University of Foggia, Foggia, Italy

Dinesh Bhugra

Emeritus Professor of Mental Health and Cultural Diversity, Health Service and Population Research Department, Institute of Psychiatry, King's College London, UK

OXFORD
UNIVERSITY PRESS

OXFORD
UNIVERSITY PRESS

Great Clarendon Street, Oxford, OX2 6DP,
United Kingdom

Oxford University Press is a department of the University of Oxford.
It furthers the University's objective of excellence in research, scholarship,
and education by publishing worldwide. Oxford is a registered trade mark of
Oxford University Press in the UK and in certain other countries

First Edition Published in 2019

Impression: 1

Published in the United States of America by Oxford University Press
198 Madison Avenue, New York, NY 10016, United States of America

British Library Cataloguing in Publication Data

Data available

Library of Congress Control Number: 2018966984

ISBN 978–0–19–882083–3

Printed and bound by
CPI Group (UK) Ltd, Croydon, CR0 4YY

Foreword

A recurring theme in the recent literature on a variety of mental disorders has been that they often remain unrecognized and untreated for a long time, not unusually several years, after the occurrence of their initial manifestations. For some disorders—such as bipolar disorder and schizophrenia—clinical research has directly documented the average interval between their onset and the time of their diagnosis and the start of appropriate treatment. For depressive disorders, a different way to document the same phenomenon has been the finding that a high proportion of cases are missed by general practitioners, although some are recognized in subsequent consultations. For other conditions—especially eating disorders and substance use disorders—the main focus has been on the multiple barriers to help-seeking, which often delay detection and treatment. In the case of Alzheimer's disease, neurobiological and neuropsychological research has been decisive in documenting the latency between the first manifestations of the illness and the clinical diagnosis.

The argument underlying this vast and diverse body of literature has been that early diagnosis and management of mental disorders may be essential in improving their course and outcome, and in reducing or even preventing their social consequences. This hypothesis has received, up until now, only partial empirical support for most of the aforementioned disorders, but represents a major focus of research for virtually all of them. Furthermore, it has been repeatedly pointed out that the reconstruction of the early phases of development of mental disorders may contribute significantly to the elucidation of their etiopathogenesis and, at least in the case of some of the disorders, may allow for the devising of prevention programmes. Recent attempts to describe a staging in the development of schizophrenia and bipolar disorder are emblematic in this respect.

This latter line of research has also helped to highlight that the expression 'early detection and management' may actually have two different meanings: on the one hand, it may refer to the timely identification and treatment of the first episode of a mental disorder; on the other, to the identification and management of those people who are at risk or at high risk, or show the 'prodromal' features of that disorder, with the aim to prevent the 'transition' to the full-blown syndrome. Early detection and management in the former sense represents, today, an undisputed target of mental health services, and the awareness is growing that the way the first episode of psychiatric illness is dealt with is also decisive in shaping the attitudes of the patient and his or her carers to psychiatric services and treatments. More controversial remains the feasibility and cost effectiveness of early detection and management in the latter sense. The recent debate on the proposal to include, in the main body of the *DSM-5*, the condition called 'attenuated psychosis syndrome' has revealed widespread concerns about the risk of false-positive diagnoses (especially in community settings), of stigmatization, and of inappropriate use of antipsychotic medications. It has been observed that teachers may view people in a different light if they carry that diagnosis, even if their behaviour is acceptable, and may consequently limit opportunities and reduce challenges. Even the family may cease to encourage growth, progress, and achievement; and there may be an impact on how the person views him or herself and makes plans for the future. There may also be consequences for obtaining insurance, especially life or disability insurance. On the other hand, the real effectiveness of the management tools available to address these 'prodromal' states has been questioned.

Furthermore, it has been observed that the current focus on 'attenuated' symptoms of a given mental disorder (such as schizophrenia) as its 'prodromal' manifestations may actually be unwarranted, because the prodromal phase may be often marked by a predominance of non-specific, fluid, and undifferentiated manifestations of emotional, cognitive, and/or behavioural dysregulation, substance abuse, family conflict, anger, tension, and low self-esteem. This line of thought has emphasized the need for a 'soft entry point' to mental health services for adolescents, aiming to intercept this fluid and undifferentiated phase, with the active involvement of young volunteers and strong support by the local community, and with a positive declared objective of educational and vocational assistance, promotion of physical and mental health, and socialization. This soft entry point could then be linked to more specific services for the more differentiated syndromes, when they begin to manifest.

The present volume summarizes the recent progress and the current challenges of this rapidly growing area of practice and research. It has the uncommon feature of covering a vast range of mental disorders, including not only psychoses and bipolar disorder—which have been the focus of literally hundreds of papers and books in recent years—but also more neglected conditions such as personality disorders and harmful alcohol use. Additionally, it covers a spectrum of approaches, from the possible contribution of brain imaging to the detection of at-risk cases, to the pathways of care for minority ethnic groups, to the different scenarios related to cultural, geographic, and health-care organization factors.

We hope that the book will be perused not only by researchers and scholars, but also by a wide range of clinicians—hopefully including also general practitioners, whose role in this area is crucial—as well as by a proportion of users and carers, who may find here better-quality and more reliable information than they can obtain from several popular websites.

Mario Maj
Past President, World Psychiatric Association

Acknowledgements

We would like to thank the staff of the Hong Kong College of Psychiatrists for helping to host the round table. Thanks are due to Sabrina Hung for her support and assistance, and also to all the authors who committed to the project both by attending the meeting and contributing, on time, in spite of their busy schedules.

Contents

Abbreviations

AAO	age at onset
AD	antidepressant
ADHD	attention deficit/hyperactivity disorder
A&E	accident and emergency
AP	antipsychotic
APS	attenuated psychotic symptoms
ARMS	at-risk mental state
ASD	autism spectrum disorder
BAR	bipolar at-risk
BASICS	Brief Alcohol Screening and Intervention for College Students
BDNF	brain-derived neurotrophic factor
B(L)IPS	brief (limited) intermittent psychotic symptoms
BOLD	Blood Oxygen Level-Dependent imaging MRI
BPD	borderline personality disorder
BS	basic symptom
CAT	cognitive analytic therapy
CBT	cognitive behaviour therapy
CHAT	community health assessment team
CJA	criminal justice agency
CRP	C-reactive protein
COGDIS	cognitive disturbance
COPER	cognitive-perceptive basic symptoms
CT	computed tomography
CUI	Clinical Utility Index
DALY	disability-adjusted life year
DBT	dialectical behaviour therapy
DSM	Diagnostic Statistical Manual
DTI	diffusion tensor imaging
DUB	duration of untreated bipolar
DUI	duration of untreated illness
DUP	duration of untreated psychosis
EEG	electroencephalography
EI(S)	early intervention (services)
EPIP	early psychosis intervention programme
ERP	event related potential
ET-BD	early transition to BD
FA	fractional anisotropy
FEP	first-episode psychosis
FFT	family-focused treatment
GABA	gamma-aminobutyric acid
GAF	global assessment of functioning
GBD	global burden of disease
GM	grey matter
GP	general practitioner
GWAS	genome-wide association
HCL	hypomania checklist
HED	heavy episodic drinking
IPSRT	interpersonal social rhythm therapy
LTD	long-term depression
LTP	long-term potentiation
PFA	psychological first aid
MBT	mentalization-based therapy
MDD	major depressive disorder
MDQ	Mood Disorders Questionnaire
MHC	major histocompatibility
MHG	mental health gap
MRC-SDS	Medical Research Council Sociodemographic Schedule
(f)MRI	(functional) magnetic resonance imaging
MRS	magnetic resonance spectroscopy
NIH	National Institute of Health
NNS	number needed to screen

NOS	not otherwise specified
OPD	outpatient department
OSBD	offspring of parents with BD
OTP	optimal treatment project
PD	personality disorder
PET	positron emission tomography
PNN	perineuronal net
PPHS	personal and psychiatric history schedule
SAPS	scale for assessment of positive symptoms
SAS	social adjustment scale
SBI	screening and brief intervention
SCID	structured clinical interview for DSM-IV-TR
SIPS	structured interview for psychosis-risk syndromes
SPI(A)/(CY)	schizophrenia proneness instrument (adult)/(child/youth)
SQL	structured query language
SSRI	selective serotonin reuptake inhibitor
TCM	traditional Chinese medicine
TEAS	treatment-emergent affective switch
tES	transcranial electrical stimulation
TMS	transcranial magnetic stimulation
UHR	ultra-high risk
UP	unipolar disorder
VEGF	vascular endothelial growth factor
VLMT	verbal learning and memory test
WHO	World Health Organization
WM	white matter

Contributors

Arthur Guerra de Andrade
Program of the Interdisciplinary Group of Studies on Alcohol and Drugs, Department and Institute of Psychiatry, School of Medicine, University of São Paulo, São Paulo/SP, Brazil

Dinesh Bhugra
Emeritus Professor of Mental Health and Cultural Diversity, Health Service and Population Research Department, Institute of Psychiatry, King's College London, UK

Sherry Kit-wa Chan
Clinical Assistant Professor, Department of Psychiatry, University of Hong Kong, Queen Mary Hospital, Hong Kong, China

Andrew Chanen
Orygen, The National Centre of Excellence in Youth Mental Health, Victoria, Australia
Centre for Youth Mental Health, The University of Melbourne, Melbourne, Australia

Wing-chung Chang
Clinical Assistant Professor, Department of Psychiatry, University of Hong Kong, Queen Mary Hospital, Hong Kong, China

Eric Y.H. Chen
Head and Professor, Department of Psychiatry, University of Hong Kong, Queen Mary Hospital, Hong Kong, China

Eric Fuk-chi Cheung
Castle Peak Hospital, Hong Kong, China

Catherine Shiu-yin Chong
Department of Psychiatry, Kwai Chung Hospital, Hong Kong, China

Dicky Wai-sau Chung
Chief of Service and Consultant, Department of Psychiatry, Alice Ho Miu Ling Nethersole Hospital, Tai Po Hospital, North District Hospital, Hong Kong, China

Tom K.J. Craig
Health Service and Population Research, Institute of Psychiatry, Psychology and Neuroscience, King's College London, UK

Carla Dalbosco
Center for Drug and Alcohol Research, Clinics Hospital of Porto Alegre, Federal University of Rio Grande do Sul, Porto Alegre/RS, Brazil

Paulina do Carmo Arruda Vieira Duarte
Department of Public Security of the Secretariat for Multidimensional Security, Organization of American States, Washington, DC, USA

Peter Falkai
Department of Psychiatry and Psychotherapy, Hospital of the University of Munich, Germany

Tomoyuki Funatogawa
Department of Neuropsychiatry, Toho University Faculty of Medicine, Tokyo, Japan

Telma Tiemi Schwindt Diniz Gomes
Center for Information on Health and Alcohol (CISA), São Paulo/SP, Brazil

Amber Hamilton
Department of Psychiatry, Faculty of Medicine and Health, Northern Clinical School, The University of Sydney, CADE Clinic, Royal North Shore Hospital Sydney, New South Wales, Australia

Christy Lai-ming Hui
Assistant Professor, Department of Psychiatry, University of Hong Kong, Queen Mary Hospital, Hong Kong, China

Naomi Inoue
Department of Neuropsychiatry, Toho University Faculty of Medicine, Tokyo, Japan

Srividya Iyer
Prevention and Early Intervention Program for Psychosis, Douglas Mental Health University Institute, Verdun, Canada

Naoyuki Katagiri
Department of Neuropsychiatry, Toho University Faculty of Medicine, Tokyo, Japan

Matcheri S. Keshavan
Beth Israel Deaconess Medical Center, Department of Psychiatry, and Harvard Medical School Department of Psychiatry, Boston, USA

Nikolaos Koutsouleris
Department of Psychiatry and Psychotherapy, Hospital of the University of Munich, Germany

Edwin Ho-ming Lee
Assistant Professor, Department of Psychiatry, University of Hong Kong, Queen Mary Hospital, Hong Kong, China

Helen Lee
Deputy Head and Principal Case Manager,
Early Psychosis Intervention Programme at the Department of Psychosis, Institute of Mental Health, Singapore

Paulo Lizano
Beth Israel Deaconess Medical Center, Department of Psychiatry, and Harvard Medical School Department of Psychiatry, Boston, USA

Tak-lam Lo
Department of Psychiatry, Kwai Chung Hospital, Hong Kong, China

Poon Lye Yin
Senior Manager, Operations, Institute of Mental Health, Singapore

Gin S. Malhi
Department of Psychiatry, Faculty of Medicine and Health, Northern Clinical School, The University of Sydney, CADE Clinic, Royal North Shore Hospital Sydney, New South Wales, Australia

Ashok Malla
Prevention and Early Intervention Program for Psychosis, Douglas Mental Health University Institute, Verdun, Canada

Masafumi Mizuno
Department of Neuropsychiatry, Toho University Faculty of Medicine, Tokyo, Japan

Greeshma Mohan
Project Coordinator, Schizophrenia Research Foundation, Chennai, India

Craig Morgan
Health Service and Population Research, Institute of Psychiatry, Psychology and Neuroscience, King's College London, UK

Grace Morris
Department of Psychiatry, Faculty of Medicine and Health, Northern Clinical School, The University of Sydney, CADE Clinic, Royal North Shore Hospital Sydney, New South Wales, Australia

Takahiro Nemoto
Department of Neuropsychiatry, Toho University Faculty of Medicine, Tokyo, Japan

Roger Man-kin Ng
Senior Medical Officer, Department of Psychiatry, Kwai Chung Hospital, Hong Kong, China

Sherifat Oduola
Health Service and Population Research, Institute of Psychiatry, Psychology and Neuroscience, King's College London, UK

John M. Oldham
Distinguished Emeritus Professor, Menninger Department of Psychiatry and Behavioral Sciences, Baylor College of Medicine, Houston, Texas, USA

Tim Outhred
Department of Psychiatry, Faculty of Medicine and Health, Northern Clinical School, The University of Sydney, CADE Clinic, Royal North Shore Hospital Sydney, New South Wales, Australia

Jaya Padmanabhan
Beth Israel Deaconess Medical Center, Department of Psychiatry, and Harvard Medical School Department of Psychiatry, Boston, USA

R. Padmavati
Director, Schizophrenia Research Foundation, Chennai, India

Lap-tak Poon
Department of Psychiatry, Kwai Chung Hospital, Hong Kong, China

Megan Pope
Prevention and Early Intervention Program for Psychosis, Douglas Mental Health University Institute, Verdun, Canada

Moritz Rossner
Department of Psychiatry and Psychotherapy, Hospital of the University of Munich, Germany

Norman Sartorius
Association for the Improvement of Mental Health Programmes, Geneva, Switzerland

Andrea Schmitt
Department of Psychiatry and Psychotherapy, Hospital of the University of Munich, Germany

Frauke Schultze-Lutter
Department of Psychiatry and Psychotherapy, Medical Faculty, Heinrich-Heine University, Düsseldorf, Germany

Thomas Schulze
Department of Psychiatry and Psychotherapy, Hospital of the University of Munich, Germany

Jan Scott
Professor of Psychological Medicine, Academic Psychiatry, Institute of Neuroscience, Newcastle University, Newcastle-upon-Tyne, UK

Chong Siow Ann
Professor, Senior Consultant Psychiatrist, Institute of Mental Health, Singapore

Erica Rosanna Siu
Program of the Interdisciplinary Group of Studies on Alcohol and Drugs, Department and Institute of Psychiatry, School of Medicine, University of São Paulo, São Paulo/SP, Brazil

R. Thara
Vice Chairman and Chair, Research and DEMCARES, Schizophrenia Research Foundation, Chennai, India

Naohisa Tsujino
Department of Neuropsychiatry, Toho University Faculty of Medicine, Tokyo, Japan

Antonio Ventriglio
Psychiatrist, Department of Mental Health, Department of Clinical and Experimental Medicine, University of Foggia, Foggia, Italy

Swapna K. Verma
Associate Professor, Chief, Department of Psychosis and East Region, Institute of Mental Health, Singapore
Clinical Assistant Dean, Duke-NUS Medical School, Singapore

Wai-song Yeung
Department of Psychiatry, Kwai Chung Hospital, Hong Kong, China

Chapter 1

Introduction

Eric Y.H. Chen, Antonio Ventriglio, and Dinesh Bhugra

Historical background of early intervention in psychiatry

The concept of early intervention (EI) has always been a general principle in medicine, including psychiatry. The fact that there is a relative lack of emphasis on early intervention for psychiatric disorders until the mid 1990s is itself noteworthy [1]. It is illuminating to understand the wider context within which psychiatric service development has evolved and in which early intervention efforts have emerged more recently, as an important direction for service development.

A recent historical review observed that discussions of early intervention for 'incipient insanity' were in fact not neglected in the literature of the second half of the nineteenth century [2]. From these discussions, it can also be observed that the difficulties confronting the early proponents of EI were in many ways similar to those of the twenty-first century—namely, the lack of an optimal means to identify the disorders in their very early stages, as well as the lack of appropriate treatment settings.

The perceived roles of mental hospitals (asylums) in the nineteenth century were associated with involuntary detention of people with severe mental disorders. Towards the end of the nineteenth century, the conditions in many asylums were overcrowded and quality of care unappealing. They became treatment settings for crisis precipitated by severe illness, in which few alternatives existed. However, they were not suitable platforms for engaging people in the earliest 'incipient' stages, with milder symptoms, for whom the need for treatment was perceived to be less pressing [2]. Thus, from the earliest days, the possibility of EI has been inextricably linked with the setting and quality of care. Modern EI proponents should not be blind to this historical lesson. In order to involve people in the earlier stages of disturbance, intervention needs to be conducted in a more positive and engaging setting [3]. From this perspective, it is also not difficult to understand how, in the context of high stigma and negative perception of psychiatric treatments, the lack of opportunity for EI extended even into the second half of the twentieth century, long after effective pharmacotherapies and psychotherapy for many psychiatric disorders had already been introduced.

The situation with psychotic disorders, for example schizophrenia, offers an illustration. Since the description of the condition as dementia praecox by Kraepelin, the expectation that patients with schizophrenia invariably progress towards a poor outcome has been a pervasive but unchallenged assumption in psychiatric circles [4–6]. More recently, with increasing emphasis on the brain mechanisms underlying psychosis (e.g. genetics and brain-structure findings), negative expectations have been further consolidated through a generally deterministic view of how genes and brain structures influence behaviour in a one-way manner [7]. Genetics and brain-imaging findings were inadvertently reinforced by a neurodevelopmental research paradigm which proposed that early brain development largely determines the onset and outcome of psychosis [8]. This perspective assumed that severe impairments were already present before the onset of illness, to an extent similar to the level of impairment eventually reached in chronic patients [9–11]. This paradigm thus reinforced a highly deterministic view of the course of psychiatric disorders. Chronicity and disability became expected outcomes, with little possibility of prevention and intervention. According to this perspective, a diagnosis of schizophrenia was similar to that of an incurable disorder, in which little could be done to modify its course. This negative view did not encourage early detection or intervention.

In the latter half of the twentieth century, the emergence of community psychiatry enabled more efforts to relocate patients from psychiatric hospitals to a community treatment setting. A new generation of outcome studies had allowed the observation of the progression of illness without the complication of institutionalization [12–15]. These studies revealed a more hopeful outcome, in that a significant proportion of patients with severe mental illness could make a good recovery.

With the increasing availability of community outcome data, the important observation was made that for psychotic disorders, poor outcome was often associated with a long delay before receiving effective treatment (duration of untreated psychosis, DUP) [16–19]. With the advent of semi-structured measurement of the DUP [20], this relationship was confirmed in many studies. It was also noticed that the DUP was relatively lengthy in many cohorts (mean 1–2 years), including those from populations enjoying well-developed community psychiatric services [5, 21, 22]. This observation opened up the question of whether shortening the delays to receiving treatment could modify the outcome [23–25].

Early proponents of EI [1, 26–28] started to articulate a set of initiatives—comprising early detection as well as specific intervention programmes—to promote the early identification and treatment of psychotic illnesses. Focusing specific intervention on the early stages of the illness was encouraged by the 'critical period hypothesis' which proposed that there is an early window of time in which the outcomes for individual illness are relatively open to modification, but after which, they become more fixed and determined [29]. The critical period hypothesis was suggested following the observation that long-term outcome was largely determined by outcomes in the first few years [30–34]. This knowledge provided a rationale for EI programmes to focus effort on the early years in the course of the disorder. Notwithstanding its appeal, the critical period hypothesis needs to be confirmed by suitable long-term outcome studies.

In the 1990s, disorder-specific research led to a paradigm for studying disorder at the first presentation (first-episode studies) [6, 35]. These studies have enriched our knowledge of the presentation and treatment responses in the early stages of various psychiatric disorders. They have also facilitated the awareness of distinctive features of illness expression in the early stages. These observations have informed us that clinical knowledge from the chronic stage cannot be uncritically transferred to the early stage of a disorder. There is a need for a specialized approach to the early stage of a disorder, both in observation and in intervention [36]. Thus, a common paradigm for early intervention work gradually developed in the context of interacting progress in research and in service delivery [37]. Although much of the pioneering work in psychosis has been carried out in the context of psychotic disorders, the same paradigm has been applied to different disorders. Indeed, there has been a suggestion that in the very early stage of incubation of mental illnesses, symptoms may be less disorder-specific, necessitating a more generic and embracing approach.

Basic framework of early intervention programmes

Many EI programmes were initiated in an era when evidence-based medicine was coming to maturity [38–40]. The alignment of service development with research initiatives resulted in an approach that was often guided by vigorous outcome evaluation and extensive use of quantitative methodologies. The emphasis on empirical evidence has facilitated a common conceptualization of the core components in early psychosis work, which can be applied to different disorders across different settings [1].

The key components of EI work can be articulated as follows:

1. *Early detection*: the objective is to reduce the duration of untreated illness in established disorders.
2. *Phase-specific intervention*: the objective is both to provide impactful intervention in the first few years (critical period), aimed specifically at addressing challenges in the early stages of a disorder, and to improve the outcome in this critical period.
3. *Sustaining the critical-period outcome*: the expectation is that the improved outcome in the critical period can be sustained in the longer term following the withdrawal of intensive phase-specific intervention.
4. *Indicated prevention*: identifying subjects at increased risk of developing a disorder and providing interventions that could reduce its full-blown development (transition) in such at-risk populations.

The articulation of these overarching principles for early intervention provides a framework within which a variety of programmes have been implemented in different localities [41, 42]. These real-life implementations have provided important opportunities to reflect on the outcome of different approaches and how they interact with specific circumstances in specific cultural and service settings.

This book originates from a global mental health workshop on EI approaches organized by the World Psychiatric Association and the Hong Kong College of Psychiatrists. The scope of the workshop was to facilitate dialogue between international leaders in EI for different psychiatric disorders on how the general framework for EI can be applied to a wide range of mental health disorders and to different cultural and service settings.

Across different settings and disorders, a common challenge to the early presentation of psychiatric disorders is the negative stigma towards mental illness. In Chapter 2, Norman Sartorius reviews the impact of stigma on treatment of psychiatric conditions and considers the process of stigma formation, suggesting ways in which EI can be considered to address the problems of stigma. The EI approach in the broader context of global mental health efforts is considered by Antonio Ventriglio and Dinesh Bhugra in Chapter 3.

Focusing on psychotic disorders, Matcheri Keshavan and colleagues provide a comprehensive summary in Chapter 4 of recent neurobiological findings on psychotic disorders, which offers a knowledge base for informing EI strategies. In Chapter 5, Peter Falkai et al. review brain changes prior to psychosis which are relevant for formulating a preventative approach, and, in Chapter 6, Frauke Schultze-Lutter reviews, in detail, the search for ways to screen for the earliest predictive symptoms in the evolution of psychotic disorders. Sherifat

Oduola and colleagues describe, in Chapter 7, data on help-seeking in first-episode psychosis in London for minority groups, highlighting the importance of understanding ethnicity-specific patterns of presentation in multicultural settings.

The interaction between EI principles and real-life societal and service contexts is discussed in detail through a number of programmes. In Chapter 8, Eric Chen and colleagues describe the early psychosis intervention programme in Hong Kong and review a number of long-term studies associated with this programme. Through this data, it is possible to reflect on the implementation outcome of the various components in the EI approach. The comprehensive early psychosis initiative in Singapore, the evaluation of the outcomes, as well as the future plan for moving towards a broader youth mental-health approach is discussed by Swapna Verma et al. in Chapter 9. In Chapter 10, Masafumi Mizuno and colleagues review the challenges of implementing early psychosis programmes in Japan, describing complex interactions between service-delivery models, health-service funding models, as well as the implemented model in Tokyo. Greeshma Mohan and colleagues consider, in Chapter 11, the important role of family in EI for psychosis in an Indian setting, using qualitative data from cross-cultural studies on early psychosis care.

EI approaches for other disorders are also considered in depth in this book. In Chapters 12 and 13 respectively, Jan Scott and Gin Malhi et al. provide insightful considerations on the challenges encountered when applying the EI paradigm to bipolar disorders, using data from the UK as well as from Australia. The rationale and efforts to provide an EI service for people with personality disorders in the USA is reviewed by John Oldham in Chapter 14, and, for borderline personality disorder specifically, by Andrew Chanen in Chapter 15. In Chapter 16, Arthur Guerra de Andrade and colleagues provide a comprehensive overview of using the EI paradigm to address harmful alcohol use in Brazil. In Chapter 17, Bhugra et al. highlight the importance of considering culture in the delivery of early intervention services, leading to recommendations for researchers, clinicians, as well as policy makers.

The structure of the book is such that each chapter can be considered independently on its own. For those who wish to follow a more systematic approach, it may be worthwhile to start with the chapters on psychotic disorders, and then follow up with chapters on other conditions. As reflected in real-life developments, as well as this book, EI approaches have so far been applied most extensively to psychotic disorders. The concepts and experience from psychosis EI can then be profitably applied, with appropriate adaptations, to other disorders.

References

1. **McGorry PD, Edwards J, Mihalopoulos C, Harrigan SM, Jackson HJ.** EPPIC: an evolving system of early detection and optimal management. Schizophr Bull. 1996; **22**(2):305–26.
2. **Chau HS, Chong WS, Wong JG, Hung GB, Lui SS, Chan SK,** et al. Early intervention for incipient insanity: early notions from the 19th century English literature. Early Interv Psychiatry. 2018; **12**(4):708–14.
3. **McGorry PD, Hickie IB, Yung AR, Pantelis C, Jackson HJ.** Clinical staging of psychiatric disorders: a heuristic framework for choosing earlier, safer and more effective interventions. Aust NZ J Psychiatry. 2006; **40**(8):616–22.
4. **Kopelowicz A, Bidder TG.** Outcome of schizophrenia. Am J Psychiatry. 1992; **149**(3):426–7.
5. **Penttila M, Jaaskelainen E, Hirvonen N, Isohanni M, Miettunen J.** Duration of untreated psychosis as predictor of long-term outcome in schizophrenia: systematic review and meta-analysis. Br J Psychiatry. 2014; **205**(2):88–94.
6. **Perkins DO, Gu H, Boteva K, Lieberman JA.** Relationship between duration of untreated psychosis and outcome in first-episode schizophrenia: a critical review and meta-analysis. Am J Psychiatry. 2005; **162**(10):1785–804.
7. **Link BG, Yang LH, Phelan JC, Collins PY.** Measuring mental illness stigma. Schizophr Bull. 2004; **30**(3):511–41.
8. **Murray RM, Lewis SW.** Is schizophrenia a neurodevelopmental disorder? BMJ. 1987; **295**(6600):681–2.
9. **Aleman A, Hijman R, de Haan EH, Kahn RS.** Memory impairment in schizophrenia: a meta-analysis. Am J Psychiatry. 1999; **156**(9):1358–66.
10. **Harrison PJ.** The neuropathology of schizophrenia. A critical review of the data and their interpretation. Brain. 1999; **122**(Pt 4):593–624.
11. **Saykin AJ, Gur RC, Gur RE, Mozley PD, Mozley LH, Resnick SM,** et al. Neuropsychological function in schizophrenia. Selective impairment in memory and learning. Arch Gen Psychiatry. 1991; **48**(7):618–24.
12. **Harding CM, Brooks GW, Ashikaga T, Strauss JS, Breier A.** The Vermont longitudinal study of persons with severe mental illness, II: Long-term outcome of subjects who retrospectively met DSM-III criteria for schizophrenia. Am J Psychiatry. 1987; **144**(6):727–35.
13. **Harding CM, Brooks GW, Ashikaga T, Strauss JS, Breier A.** The Vermont longitudinal study of persons with severe mental illness, I: Methodology, study sample, and overall status 32 years later. Am J Psychiatry. 1987; **144**(6):718–26.
14. **McGlashan TH.** The Chestnut Lodge follow-up study. I. Follow-up methodology and study sample. Arch Gen Psychiatry. 1984; **41**(6):573–85.
15. **McGlashan TH.** The Chestnut Lodge follow-up study. II. Long-term outcome of schizophrenia and the affective disorders. Arch Gen Psychiatry. 1984; **41**(6):586–601.
16. **Craig TJ, Bromet EJ, Fennig S, Tanenberg-Karant M, Lavelle J, Galambos N.** Is there an association between duration of untreated psychosis and 24-month clinical outcome in a first-admission series? Am J Psychiatry. 2000; **157**(1):60–6.
17. **Lo WH, Lo T.** A ten-year follow-up study of Chinese schizophrenics in Hong Kong. Br J Psychiatry. 1977; **131**:63–6.

18. **Loebel AD, Lieberman JA, Alvir JM, Mayerhoff DI, Geisler SH, Szymanski SR.** Duration of psychosis and outcome in first-episode schizophrenia. Am J Psychiatry. 1992; **149**(9):1183–8.
19. **Waddington JL, Youssef HA, Kinsella A.** Sequential cross-sectional and 10-year prospective study of severe negative symptoms in relation to duration of initially untreated psychosis in chronic schizophrenia. Psychol Med. 1995; **5**(4):849–57.
20. **Hafner H, Riecher-Rossler A, Hambrecht M, Maurer K, Meissner S, Schmidtke A**, et al. IRAOS: an instrument for the assessment of onset and early course of schizophrenia. Schizophr Res. 1992; **6**(3):209–23.
21. **Boonstra N, Klaassen R, Sytema S, Marshall M, De Haan L, Wunderink L**, et al. Duration of untreated psychosis and negative symptoms–a systematic review and meta-analysis of individual patient data. Schizophr Res. 2012; **142**(1–3):12–9.
22. **Norman RM, Malla AK.** Duration of untreated psychosis: a critical examination of the concept and its importance. Psychol Med. 2001; **31**(3):381–400.
23. **Larsen TK, Friis S, Haahr U, Johannessen JO, Melle I, Opjordsmoen S**, et al. Premorbid adjustment in first-episode non-affective psychosis: distinct patterns of pre-onset course. Br J Psychiatry. 2004; **185**:108–15.
24. **McGlashan TH.** Premorbid adjustment, onset types, and prognostic scaling: still informative? Schizophr Bull. 2008; **34**(5):801–5.
25. **Melle I, Larsen TK, Haahr U, Friis S, Johannessen JO, Opjordsmoen S**, et al. Reducing the duration of untreated first-episode psychosis: effects on clinical presentation. Arch Gen Psychiatry. 2004; **61**(2):143–50.
26. **Birchwood M, McGorry P, Jackson H.** Early intervention in schizophrenia. Br J Psychiatry. 1997; **170**:2–5.
27. **McGlashan TH.** Early detection and intervention in schizophrenia: research. Schizophr Bull. 1996; **22**(2):327–45.
28. **Wyatt RJ.** Early intervention for schizophrenia: can the course of the illness be altered? Biol Psychiatry. 1995; **38**(1):1–3.
29. **Birchwood MP, Todd P, Jackson C.** Early intervention in psychosis. The critical period hypothesis. Br J Psychiatry Suppl. 1998; **172**(33):53–9.
30. **Carpenter WT**, Jr., **Strauss JS.** The prediction of outcome in schizophrenia. IV: Eleven-year follow-up of the Washington IPSS cohort. J Nerv Ment Dis. 1991; **179**(9):517–25.
31. **Eaton WW, Thara R, Federman E, Tien A.** Remission and relapse in schizophrenia: the Madras Longitudinal Study. J Nerv Ment Dis. 1998; **186**(6):357–63.
32. **Harrison G, Croudace T, Mason P, Glazebrook C, Medley I.** Predicting the long-term outcome of schizophrenia. Psychol Med. 1996; **26**(4):697–705.
33. **Thara R, Henrietta M, Joseph A, Rajkumar S, Eaton WW.** Ten-year course of schizophrenia—the Madras longitudinal study. Acta Psychiatr Scand. 1994; **90**(5):329–36.
34. **Todd NA.** First episode schizophrenia: three year and sixteen year follow-up. Health Bull. 1988; **46**(1):18–25.
35. **Mesholam-Gately RI, Giuliano AJ, Goff KP, Faraone SV, Seidman LJ.** Neurocognition in first-episode schizophrenia: a meta-analytic review. Neuropsychology. 2009; **23**(3):315–36.

36. **Mihalopoulos C, McGorry PD, Carter RC.** Is phase-specific, community-oriented treatment of early psychosis an economically viable method of improving outcome? Acta Psychiatr Scand. 1999; **100**(1):47–55.
37. **Chen EY-h, Lee H, Chan GH-k, Wong GH-y.** Early psychosis intervention: a culturally adaptive clinical guide. Hong Kong University Press; 2013.
38. **Adams CE, Fenton MK, Quraishi S, David AS.** Systematic meta-review of depot antipsychotic drugs for people with schizophrenia. Br J Psychiatry. 2001; **179**:290–9.
39. **Berk SBFNM.** Risperidone compared to haloperidol in cannabis-induced psychotic disorder: A double blind randomized controlled trial. Int J Psychiatry Clin Pract. 2000; **4**(2):139–42.
40. **Emsley R, Oosthuizen P.** Evidence-based pharmacotherapy of schizophrenia. Int J Neuropsychopharmacol. 2004; **7**(2):219–38.
41. **Edwards J, McGorry PD.** Implementing early intervention in psychosis: a guide to establishing early psychosis services. London: Martin Dunitz; 2002. p. xv, p. 186.
42. **Ehmann T, MacEwan GW, Honer WG.** Best care in early psychosis intervention: global perspectives. London, New York: Taylor & Francis; 2004.

Chapter 2

Early interventions to prevent stigmatization and its consequences

Norman Sartorius

Introduction

Mental disorders are stigmatized in all known cultures. Stigma can sometimes lead to positive consequences (persons with a mental illness may be seen by their group as being linked to the supranatural, possibly to a deity) but this is rare, and becoming rarer. Most often, stigma of mental illness makes the person who has it a subject of discrimination in all fields of life. People with mental illness are excluded from their peer groups, they have difficulties finding employment or a place to live, potential marital partners shun them, and their children are usually ashamed to have them as parents. Stigma does not end with the person who has a mental illness: it expands to the members of their family, to institutions in which they receive treatment, to medications which are used to treat them, and to health workers who provide care for them.

Stigmatization is a result of concept formation during which individuals learn to recognize the essential characteristics of a group of individuals or things that have many different characteristics. Thus the concept of 'dog' applies to a variety of animals, tall and small, aggressive and cuddly, with different forms of ears, eyes, snouts, tails, and pelts. Yet, once the concept of 'dog' is formed—perhaps characterized by the fact that all dogs bark—this variety of characteristics can be disregarded, which simplifies the child's relationship with the world. People with mental illness have as their common characteristic that their behaviour is not as predictable as that of other humans, and thus members of the community label them as mentally ill or abnormal, and avoid them as they would avoid an alien who is unpredictable and potentially dangerous. If they are unlikely to be dangerous, for example because they are physically feeble and clumsy, they will, in many cultures, become subjects of ridicule or exploitation: by being both avoided and teased, they are shown to be considered less valuable than people without mental illness [1].

Concept formation begins early in life and becomes less intensive as children grow up and become adults. The world in which adults live is comprehensible and describable because concept formation has simplified it. The immense number of things and beings that surrounds an adult has been reduced, condensed by ordering the variety of phenomena into concepts. Without such concepts it is difficult to function. Humans are very reluctant to 'undo' concepts and reorder things, events, or beings into new concepts because the reorganization of concepts is logically accompanied by uncertainty, lesser competence, and poorer performance, thus creating a period of enhanced danger.

One of the consequences of this way of growing into the world and surviving in it is that efforts to reduce the stigma of mental illness must begin very early, in childhood—in time to prevent the creation of the concept of the mad person characterized by features such as unpredictability, dangerousness, clumsiness, and incomprehensible behaviour, and as being less human than the rest and best avoided or eliminated from society.

Participants in early interventions against stigma of mental disorders

Parents, members of the community, other children, and headlines and reports in the media are the first to influence children in the formation of concepts. They do this by what they say and by what they do, often unaware of the influence that they have on the process of concept formation. It is not possible to control all the influences that reach the child, but some are amenable to adjustment. The behaviour of parents when they encounter a disabled person is observed, retained, and often imitated by children. The comments about other people's behaviour are remembered by children and used in the process of concept formation.

Education for parenthood can be low in cost and short in duration. It does not require special facilities nor huge additional resources, and yet it can have a profound influence on the mental health of parents and their life, as well as on the life and social networking of their children. It is a significantly neglected opportunity to contribute to the improvement of mental health and to the creation of a better society. It gains in importance by the increasing number of children living with one of the parents and with the decreasing opportunities to learn from elders and family members usually surrounding children in rural and traditional family settings. Education for parenthood can help parents to establish a better relationship with their children. It can also alert parents to the unconscious transmission of positions and attitudes, including those of relationships with people who have a mental illness and other social relationships which the future adult will establish and should maintain. Yet, education for parenthood is rarely if ever monitored in describing strategies to reduce or to prevent stigma [2].

Schools are places in which children, and then adolescents, may have spent 15,000 hours by the end of their teens. The curricula that govern these hours dictate the broad range of subjects that children study and describe the knowledge that they should acquire during their time in school. Thus, children may well leave school able, for example, to list the kings of various countries, to understand elementary chemical reactions, having mastered basic manipulations of simple and higher mathematics, or having read classical works of literature. However, the curricula do not specify how children should acquire the skills of conversation and other social skills which will be undoubtedly useful in later life, and perhaps help them more than factual knowledge. They do not specify how children should learn to live with people who are of a different culture, handicapped, impaired in some way, or mentally unwell. The system of education in which adolescents and young adults are living on university campuses is even worse because it places young people into an unreal world in which there are no elderly, no invalids, no drunkards, no poor people, and no people with illnesses that diminish their capacity and make them behave in the ways of people who are not well. At the end of their university or college days, students often have fine intentions and a lot of knowledge, but little experience of life and relationships with the various members of their own or other communities.

Media such as radio, television, and the press have been shown to contribute to the formation of attitudes. Being, on the whole, committed to the presentation of sensational material, media often link violence, heartlessness, cruelty, and similar features with mental illness and, thus, contribute to the formation of both negative attitudes to mental illness and to its stigma. In some instances—for example, in Ireland and in the Philippines—journalists have reached agreements about the way in which they will write or speak about mental illness and people with mental disorders so as to avoid stigmatization and the creation of negative attitudes to mentally-ill people. In many other settings, this has not happened and media do contribute to the creation and maintenance of stigma [3].

Legislation concerning people with mental illness (and other legislation) often reflects, and supports, the attitudes of the public. This creates a vicious circle in which negative attitudes of the public guide the development of prejudicial and discriminatory legislation which then supports and strengthens the negative attitudes. Many countries have adopted a mental health act to prevent the abuse of human rights of the mentally ill and to protect the citizens from dangerous acts that may occur as a consequence of mental illness. These acts can play a useful role if used in the right way; yet, their very existence confirms discrimination on the grounds of mental illness, and it would therefore be preferable to include appropriate regulations in the general legislation which govern the behaviour of people and the protection of society against dangers that might emerge because of actions of any citizen, with or without mental illness. Even when the legal provisions concerning people with mental illness are well done, they can eventually also become obsolete, and it is essential that they include a 'sunset clause'—an obligation to review them in the light of the development of both science and society. 'Sunset clauses' are, however, only rarely found in the legislation concerning people with mental illness.

Health services are one of the sources of stigmatization of mental illness and people who have it. General hospitals often refuse to house a department of psychiatry or, if they do, they place it in a remote corner of the hospital compound, sending a powerful message that mentally-ill people are not medically ill and that it is necessary to separate them from the rest of the population. Even when a department of psychiatry is placed in the building of the hospital, it is usually hidden away in the lower ground floor. Health-care workers are not better—psychiatrists and staff of psychiatric departments, as well as personnel working in other departments, are a powerful source of stigmatization without being aware of this. The language used to describe the mentally ill in ordinary conversation among health-care professionals reflects their prejudices and influences the general public. Complaints about pain or other problems brought forward by people with mental illness are given considerably less attention than the same complaints expressed by other patients. People with mental illness are given fewer laboratory examinations when they have a physical illness, and the care which they receive for it is inferior in quality and quantity when compared with the care for other people with the same physical illness. The mortality of mentally-ill people is much higher than the mortality from the same diseases in people who do not have a mental illness, and the main reason for this is the neglect of care both by those with mental illness and by health services which serve them.

Principles of interventions to reduce stigma and discrimination because of mental illness

In view of differences in the manner in which stigma reflects itself, and the variety of cultural and subcultural settings in which stigma should be fought, it is necessary to recognize that programmes against stigma will be different from one another and that their success will have to be measured by different indicators.

The decisions about the way in which a programme should be developed are often reached after an examination of the evidence obtained by studies carried out in one's own country—or, if these have not been undertaken, using evidence obtained in other countries. Experience has, however, shown that programmes built on the basis of research often fail to achieve their goals and that those most concerned—people with mental illness and their families—are not particularly keen to participate in such programmes. This is not difficult to understand: studies usually assemble data on representative samples of the population and disregard small but significant differences among population groups and subgroups. Thus, while scientific investigations are informative in matters concerning the causes and determinants of stigmatization, they are too general to evoke the enthusiastic support of population groups which identify themselves only partially with the average 'representative' findings. Programmes against stigma must therefore be built on data directly obtained from the groups of the population which are to benefit from interventions. If action is directed at problems identified locally by users of psychiatric services and caregivers, it will receive their support and commitment to participate in further joint activities.

Focusing on locally identified problems—building a programme, like a mosaic, in which different localities have slightly different centres of attention (and of action)—does not prevent (nor should it) action on a global or national level (e.g. to change legislation or insurance rules). An advantage of this model—of some action at central level plus a variety of locally relevant activities—is that it generates examples of successful programmes, which not only encourage all concerned but also offer options for further involvement [4].

Another paradigm of fighting stigma which requires revisiting is that of the need to develop precise, long-term anti-stigma programmes. It is only rarely possible to develop realistic plans which govern action over a long period of time. Plans should therefore contain only a few general principles and rules, and have provisions to enable programmes to use opportunities for anti-stigma action as they arise. This strategy of 'enlightened opportunism' may not be very attractive to potential funders and government officials engaged in building long-term perspectives and activities—yet it is more likely to bring success. The fact that the president or health minister of a country has a mentally-ill relative will, as a rule, make them more approachable and more interested in building programmes concerned with mental illness and related stigma or discrimination—but, in most countries, it is not possible to foresee when such persons will be elected to high office. It is therefore necessary to develop anti-stigma programmes with the capacity to change direction in order to follow an opportunity, rather than insist on programmes which are logical and clear but exist in a vacuum, unconcerned with the reality in which they have to be implemented.

An often-used strategy of anti-stigma programmes is the education of the general public about mental illnesses— their causes, their forms, and their frequency. This strategy is based on the notion that people who have sufficient knowledge about mental illness will be less prejudiced and more likely to include mentally-ill persons in their midst. Unfortunately, research and experience show that this is not the case. Health literacy is useful—for example, in disease-prevention programmes—but it does not diminish stigma nor discrimination. The main reason for this is probably the selective memory and perception usually accompanying prejudice: of all the information provided in educational programmes, those that are prejudiced will remember that which confirms their prejudice and will quickly forget that which is not harmonious with their prejudice.

Anti-stigma programmes sometimes rely on campaigns (e.g. devoting a day, a month, or a year to action against stigma). Such campaigns have been shown to be useful if they are occasional paroxysms of a permanent programme against stigma—a programme that is an integral part of a mental health or public health service. If they are no more than occasional events, they have little effect and often leave people with mental illness, and their families, bitter when they stop because there is no follow-up to the emphasis and activities that marked the campaign.

The considerations mentioned earlier exemplify ways in which strategies that have been thought to be particularly useful and desirable have had to be revised and changed in recent years. Almost none of the paradigms that were considered as being self-evident and useful can be recommended for general use: rather, the general conclusion from experience gained in building programmes is that the fight against stigma requires not only a critical appraisal of strategies that were previously recommended but also a constant readiness to evaluate and change plans in accordance with the results of the evaluation [5].

Concluding remarks

In view of the fact that stigmatization has its origin in the process of concept formation—conceiving that the common characteristic of all people with mental illness is that they are unpredictable and often incomprehensible—which begins in early childhood (using information obtained through family, community members, and media), it is of crucial importance to concentrate anti-stigma activities in childhood and early adolescence. Action concerning stigma in adulthood—once the concept of mentally-ill people is formed—will have to be mainly on fighting discrimination which is the consequence of stigmatization.

It is, of course, possible and desirable to take action which will help to reconceptualize the group of people with mental illness as being people like ourselves, yet burdened by an illness rather than being basically different. The expression 'alien' (which is used to describe a mentally-ill person) and 'alienist' (to describe a psychiatrist) is related to the behaviour of mentally-ill people who act in a manner that would be expected from people belonging to some other culture, some other planet: the change of the determining features of the concept of mental illness and the mentally ill will, therefore, have to include gradual decomposition of the concept (e.g. by demonstrating the vast differences in the way mental illness can express itself) and the introduction of different descriptors. Such a reconceptualization will take a considerable amount of time and effort, and might, in the end, have only insignificant results: hence the need to concentrate on the prevention of stigmatization in childhood and the fight against discrimination as the main activities of anti-stigma programmes.

This change of strategy is not the only one: other ways of acting and building programmes, which were developed in the past, will also have to be re-examined and reformulated if they are to be useful.

References

1. **Callard F, Sartorius N, Arboleda-Flórez J, Barlett P, Helmchen H, Stuart H,** et al., editors. Mental illness, discrimination and the law. Fighting for social justice. Chichester: Wiley-Blackwell; 2012.
2. **Rüsch N, Xu Z.** Strategies to reduce mental illness stigma. In: **Gaebel W, Rössler W, Sartorius N**, editors. The stigma of mental illness: end of the story. Switzerland: Springer International; 2017. p. 451–68.
3. **Andrade Loch A, Rössler W.** Who is Contributing? In: **Gaebel W, Rössler W, Sartorius N**, editors. The stigma of mental illness: end of the story. Switzerland: Springer International; 2017. p. 111–2.
4. **Sartorius N, Schulze H.** Reducing the stigma of mental illness. Cambridge: Cambridge University Press; 2005.
5. **Stuart H, rboleda Flores J, Sartorius N.** Paradigms lost. Oxford and New York: Oxford University Press; 2012.

Chapter 3

The role of culture in early interventions

Antonio Ventriglio and Dinesh Bhugra

Introduction

We are all—no matter where we are born—born *into* a culture, not *with* a culture. The way we are brought up follows the child-rearing patterns of that particular culture. In turn, these patterns go on to influence our social as well as cognitive development, shaping our view of the world. Such components of cognitive and social development affect the way we express distress, whether it is physical or mental or a mixture of the two. Cultures determine what is normal behaviour and what is seen as deviant. Of the three broad components of mental illness—abnormal mood, thought, or behaviour—the first two (changes in mood or thought) are about very personal experiences which may or may not be seen as abnormal by others within the individual's circle. However, abnormal behaviour will be defined and identified as 'abnormal' as seen by cultured values.

Definitions

It is important to identify what is meant by the term 'culture' so that clinicians are aware of what the impact may be. Individuals imbibe culture as they grow, develop, live, and work. Culture provides the basic framework which allows the individual to develop socially and cognitively. Child-rearing patterns are crucial in this context.

Culture can be defined as learned—not genetically inherited—shared meanings of symbols [1], which are embedded in language, rituals, religion, food, and so on. Culture consists of various aspects which contribute to the identity of the individual and defines them to a degree. It must be recognized that cultures remain heterogeneous, and are dynamic and change in response to individuals; and, in turn, individuals change in response to culture. Globalization and a resulting increase in urbanization can further contribute to what is described as acculturation. Acculturation is the process by which the groups' and individual's cultural values change.

Micro-identities contribute to an individual's overall cultural identity. These micro-identities are related to age, gender, religion, sexual orientation, and social and economic status [2]. In addition, clinicians may also carry their cultural micro-identities, which are strongly influenced by the place in which they trained and the culture of the place where they work. The therapeutic interaction thus involves two different sets of micro-identities which may be in conflict and hamper therapeutic alliance. Therefore, the culture of the clinician (and the clinic) could lead to either strained or positive interactions with their patients.

Explanatory models

Patients and their carers have an explanatory model which, to them, explains their experience of distress. The contents of the explanatory model are illustrated in Box 3.1.

Kleinman [3] proposed that understanding the patient's concept and explanations of his or her illness is the first key step to forming a therapeutic alliance. The comparison between the patient's model (which may well be supernatural or natural) and the doctor's explanatory model (which is likely to be medical or physiological) will ensure that any discrepancy between the two can be

Box 3.1 Patients' explanatory model of their experience of distress

1. What do you think is wrong with you?
2. What do you think caused it?
3. Why now?
4. What impact does it have on you?
5. How does it affect your functioning?
6. What do you think is needed?
7. Who should provide it?
8. What would you like to happen as a result?
9. What are the major problems you want resolved?
10. What do you fear most about your illness?

minimized and better improved therapeutic interactions may occur. Such an exploration may lead the doctor to find out what type of education may be required. The differences between the two models are often understood to be extreme, although there can be a major degree of overlap; or an agreement can be reached so that the two models can come together. The explanatory model is not dissimilar to the model of 'insight', but is more accommodating of patient expectations of treatment and outcomes.

The challenge for the clinician is to explore and understand what the patient is really thinking without showing prejudice or appearing patronizing. Any questions must be asked sensitively and carefully. Health beliefs of patients and their carers will also demonstrate the locus of control—whether it is external or internal. Such beliefs inevitably influence the type of treatment sought and the degree of congruence between the doctor's and the patient's models.

Disease versus illness

Eisenberg [4] observed that disease meant literally 'dis-ease', which focuses on pathology. The social impact of disease affects the functioning of the patient, and the patient recognizes it as illness. Doctors are trained to deal with disease and pathology, whereas patients are interested in getting better and dealing with their illness. The latter, according to Eisenberg [4], deal with devalued changes in the state of being and in social functioning, which means that individuals who experience illness are more likely to seek help from folk or faith healers. Contemporary medical practice has become technical and distant [5], and current psychiatric practice is in a perilous state in following that model. Illness includes the meaning given to the experience of distress by individuals, their carers, and their families. Experience of illness can be naturalistic or normative [6], which must influence the descriptions of lived experience; and training must focus on this.

Perceptions of the self across cultures: the role of culture in moulding the concept of personality of the individual

It is important to understand the role that culture plays in shaping the concept of the individual's personality, as this may well be one of the features which may affect not only the identification of distress but how and where help is sought. Hofstede [9] has suggested that cultures can be classified using various dimensions. Of these, socio-centric and egocentric cultures, and masculine/feminine dimensions, are important. However, not every individual in a socio-centric society is likely to be socio-centric, or egocentric in an egocentric society.

The concept of the self varies cross-culturally. Morris [10] argues that, following Harre [11], 'person' is an empirical concept that refers to beings in the collective (public realm), and 'self' is a concept acquired by individuals during the process of interactions. Morris [10] points out that the Western conception of the person is often reduced to a stereotype. His observations need some expansion. The self-structure of Western cultures has been widely described as individuated, detached, separate, and self-sufficient. Morris [10] does emphasize that a dualism between mind and body exists, and that radical individualism puts a fundamental emphasis on autonomy and appeals to an inner self and personality which are seen as distinct. However, the concept of 'Western', itself, deserves challenge.

The distinction between egocentric and socio-centric individuals is probably worth remembering. Gender plays a major role in identity, and different cultures see gender roles and gender-role expectations in different ways. Gender in socio-centric societies may play a different role as it would in masculine or feminine cultures. The concept of person varies cross-culturally according to universalism, evolutionism, and relativism [12]. These concepts obviously influence how individuals see themselves, and also how they perceive others see them. Any assessment must take into account the concept not only of the individual as a person but also of the broader persona of the culture within which he or she lives and functions.

Mind and brain across cultures

In our understanding of mind and brain across cultures, two key concepts must be recognized. The first one is the 'emic' approach which focuses on collection of data in the context of its own culture and language, in order to preserve the original meaning of the information. This is in contrast to the 'etic' approach which imposes meaning from an external cultural system. The terms 'emic' and 'etic' come from the field of linguistics and anthropology.

The concepts of brain and mind vary across cultures. Cartesian mind–body dualism, when it was described, was said to be affected by the role that the Church played: the Church was responsible for the soul, whereas doctors were supposed to take care of the body. However, although the distinction was not intended to be rigid, over the centuries it has become so [13]. Originally, Descartes [14] did say that he could obtain knowledge of himself without knowledge of his body. He went on to acknowledge that he may not have been aware of everything in his body, but that he was supposing that he was not aware that the mind possessed the power of moving the body. Damasio [15] notes that Descartes managed to persuade biologists to adopt a mechanical model, and also that thinking was allocated solely to the brain, and, thus, that thinking, and its awareness, are the real substances of being. Therefore, the brain became the thinking organ—the body did not. This is what Damasio [15] calls Descartes' error. In other, traditional healthcare systems, such as Ayurveda, mind and body are interlinked, and both are strongly influenced by external factors such as climate and environment, but also by diet and rituals and such like. Thus, these concepts affect explanatory models which, in turn, lead accordingly to help-seeking and subsequent therapeutic engagement. Cartesian dualism has led to a major division between psychiatry and physical medicine, with separate services and separate funding. In addition, patients who see their problems as somatic end up being investigated repeatedly, at a tremendous cost, while aspects of their mental-health needs are ignored completely. Damasio [15] argues that versions of Descartes' error obscure the roots of the human mind in a biologically complex but fragile organism.

Pathways into care

Gater et al. [7] highlighted the importance of pathways into care. Once individuals recognize distress and feel unwell, they then try to understand what is going on, and to not only give it a name but to also discover its cause and what may make it better. This explanatory model will then lead them to seek help from the most appropriate source. For example, a patient who thinks that the problem is caused by supernatural factors may seek help from folk or religious healers. One who thinks it is a physical problem or is causing somatic symptoms may go to see a doctor. Thus, the first step will be very much dictated by what the patient sees as having caused the problem. If that particular intervention fails, then the patient may well move on to the next source of help. It has been observed that 70–90 per cent of all illness episodes are treated in personal, folk, or social sectors, and only a minority end up in the professional sector.

Gater et al. [7], in a study from 11 countries, of over 1,554 new patients referred to psychiatric services, looked at the possible reasons for delay in help-seeking. Two observations stand out. Firstly, that where native healers were involved, this led to a major delay in seeking help from the professional sector, which in itself is not surprising, as the explanatory models may have affected the choice of help-seeking—something these authors did not explore. The second finding was that somatic problems were a common presentation to all centres. The centres in the countries which had more psychiatrists per head of population were more likely to have a pattern in which the general practitioner was key to referral and often an early contact.

In another study a few years later, in Eastern Europe, Gater et al. [8] used the same method in eight centres which shared common characteristics, in that all were in transition from predominantly institutional care to community-based healthcare. Cultures in transition often move from predominantly communist regimes to more free-market capitalist societies. New cases were approached and pathways studied. Suggestions to seek help first came from the family and carers; attempted suicide and behavioural problems (especially violent behaviour) were important factors. Whilst in one centre, 10 per cent of patients saw native healers, less than 2 per cent did in other centres; whereas in the first study [7], data from India and Pakistan showed that a native or religious healer was the first contact in many cases. It is possible that as the systems of healthcare are largely private, it may be cheaper to see a folk healer. Inevitably, those patients who went straight to services were more likely to express shorter delay, whereas, understandably, those who had somatic symptoms were more likely to experience delays. Not surprisingly, a diagnosis of schizophrenia was more likely to lead to help-seeking sooner. In East Europe, 50 per cent of patients, in six centres, approached psychiatric services directly. Thus, the cultural and healthcare systems will play a role in pathways to care, as well as explanatory models and ability to pay.

The studies on pathways into care across cultures have often focused on psychoses, due to lack of resources and seriousness of the conditions. It is difficult to ascertain where and how children with problems, those with intellectual disabilities, and those with alcohol and substance abuse go, and what the actual duration of the untreated period in many psychiatric conditions is. In many countries, those with substance abuse often end up in non-professional settings, with resulting problems in the medium to long term.

Further clear research is indicated to explore pathways of care for major psychiatric conditions, which can help identify what sources out-patients use and subsequent strategies for developing preventative and educational programmes. There are, of course, ethical issues (discussed later in this chapter) which must be borne in mind. Different stops along the pathways of care will determine what interventions may well be acceptable to patients, their carers, and their families.

Strategies for early intervention

There are many types of strategy for early intervention, and we do not propose to go into all of them here. However, we will point out some key interventions in a selected number of conditions. Of these, perhaps psychological first aid is most relevant and yet underutilized. Bhugra [16] proposes that any health policy must include psychological first aid (PFA). Birchwood and Macmillan [17] propose that early intervention must include a combination of medical and psychosocial interventions targeted at young vulnerable people, with the aim of preventing or limiting likely social, mental, and psychological deterioration. It has also been suggested that the three key elements of an early intervention strategy must include early detection of 'at risk' mental states, early treatment of psychotic states, and interventions targeted during the early phase of psychosis identified as the critical period [18].

Interestingly, Insel [19] recommends that the clinical care for psychiatry needs to resemble care in medicine, including participatory, personalized, predictive, and pre-emptive aspects. Of these, he argues that pre-emptive psychiatry and predictive aspects are the future of psychiatry. Thus, early detection and appropriate intervention are crucial in managing schizophrenia. Stafford et al. [20] found, after a systematic review, that although evidence of benefit for any specific intervention was not conclusive, it might be possible to prevent transition to the psychosis.

Tang et al. [21] reported from Hong Kong that early assessment services for young people with psychosis improved the patients' outcomes. In addition, the programme suggested that additional costs related to increased staffing and medication may be mitigated by a reduction in the duration of stay. The same group showed differences in the three-year outcome of 700 first-episode psychosis patients [22]. They reported that patients in the early intervention group had longer full-time employment, fewer days of hospitalization, less severe symptoms (both positive and negative), and lower rates of suicide.

Fowler et al. [23] reported that, in a ten-year cohort, implementation of comprehensive early intervention treatments could have a major impact on improving functional recovery. From London, Craig et al. [24] noted that patients in specialized interventions were less likely to relapse, and had lower rates of readmissions. The local population has a significant African Caribbean population, which makes this study of great interest. McGorry et al. [25] recommend a clinical staging model with three foci or stages: those who are at ultra-high risk, first episode, and the recovery or critical period. The concept of three stages can be easily applied across cultures without much difficulty. In Japan [26], similar efforts are underway.

Roberts et al. [27], in a systematic review, reported that trauma-focused cognitive behaviour therapy (CBT) within three months of a traumatic event appears to be effective. Others have reported similar findings [28]. Adolescents with borderline personality disorders had received cognitive analytic therapy for early intervention, which was found to be effective in reducing externalizing psychopathology [29]. Similar findings have emerged from early interventions in eating disorders [30].

However, cross-cultural studies in early intervention for most psychiatric disorders are lacking. We can only speculate on the reasons for this, which may include a lack of resources as a primary concern. It is inevitable that stigma may well also play a significant role in seeking help, as indeed may public mental health. The challenge for clinicians, researchers, and policy makers alike is that public mental health, early intervention, and clinical services should not be in separate silos, and need to be integrated in a pragmatic and sensible way.

Early interventions, especially when they are to be acknowledged across cultures, carry major ethical dilemmas with them, and this debate needs to be started in earnest and appropriate guidelines issued which may well fit with local cultural values and expectations. Some of these points are discussed next.

Ethical issues in defining disease

Prodrome and preclinical state are possibly retrospective. The preclinical state is often a non-state and there is a critical threshold; but then who defines the threshold in order to establish who is at risk and why they are at risk? If the risk of developing psychoses is calculated and it is false positive, the resulting anxiety, especially during the 'waiting period', is likely to create harm. Knowing about early intervention resulting from risk status can lead to stress, especially if early interventions are not available, either due to costs or to the health-care system or to policies which may not see this as possible. Furthermore, the known risk status may affect the possibility of getting health or other insurance, and may lead to personal difficulties. For example, the likelihood of getting married may be influenced by the individual's risk status of developing a psychiatric diagnosis. Testing for biomarkers may also carry with it special problems.

Cultural differences in communication between doctors and patients may well lead to tensions if the patients' or their carers' views and explanatory models are not taken into account when understanding the pathways patients take while seeking care.

Potentially, every individual is at risk of facing miscommunication—doctors may not be entirely equipped to communicate risk, nor patients and their families to interpret risk. Will future requirements focus on risk and early recognition of this treatment? It is entirely possible that ethical issues related to risk and treating non-states will become more complex and will require careful dialogue with the society. Disclosing wrong information—whether it is false positive or false negative—may well affect life chances and also contribute further to stigma. Hence, public engagement in different cultural contexts is critical. There is another aspect—relating to the mental health gap (MHG)—that needs clear and urgent management. In virtually every country around the world, the MHG remains remarkably high. To then plan services, in this context, for early intervention, or to make prodromal diagnoses, can contribute further to this gap. Thus, a clear dialogue within society, to identify ethical aspects, especially when cultures vary so much on a number of parameters including notions of confidentiality and privacy, needs to be taken into account.

Conclusions

There is no doubt that cultures influence idioms of distress—that is, explanatory models of the distress and its expression. Therefore, in low- and middle-income countries in particular, careful attention needs to be paid to exploring stigma and engaging with community leaders, and other key stakeholders, when planning any services which consist of early intervention. Early intervention can play a significant role in reducing the burden of disease, and also in better outcomes. In addition, working across disciplines may well help reduce stigma.

References

1. **Department of Health and Human Sciences** (DHHS). Mental health: culture, race and ethnicity. Rockville, MD: DHHS; 2000.
2. **Wachter M, Ventriglio A, Bhugra D.** Micro-identities, adjustment and stigma. Int J Soc Psychiatry. 2015; **61**:436–7.
3. **Kleinman A.** Patients and their healers in the context of their culture. University of California Press; 1980.
4. **Eisenberg L.** Disease and illness: distinctions between professional and popular ideas of sickness. Cult Med Psychiatry. 1977; **1**:9–23.
5. **Kleinman A, Eisenberg L, Good B.** Culture, illness and care: clinical lessons from anthropologic and cross-cultural research. Focus. 2006 Jan; **4**(1):140–9.
6. **Carel H.** Illness. Durham: Acumen; 2013.
7. **Gater R, Sousa BDAE, Barrientos G, Caraveo J, Chandrashekar CR, Dhadphale M**, et al. The pathways to psychiatric care: a cross-cultural study. Psychol Med. 1991; **21**:761–74.
8. **Gater R, Jordanova V, Maric N, Alikaj V, Bajs M, Cavic T**, et al. Pathways to psychiatric care in Eastern Europe. Br J Psychiatry. 2005; **186**:529–35.
9. **Hofstede G.** Culture's consequences. Sherman Oaks: Sage; 2001.
10. **Morris B.** Anthropology of the self. London: Pluto Press; 1994.
11. **Harré R.** Personal being: a theory for individual psychology. Oxford: Blackwell; 1983.

12. **Shweder R, Bourne EJ.** Does the concept of person vary cross-culturally? In: **Shweder RA, LeVine RA,** editors. Culture theory: essays on mind, self and emotion. Cambridge: Cambridge University Press; 1984. p. 158–99.
13. **Descartes R.** Descartes: selected philosophical writings. Cottingham J, Stoothoff R, Murdoch D, translators. Cambridge: Cambridge University Press; 1988.
14. **Descartes R.** The philosophical works of Descartes (1637). **Cottingham J, Stoothoff R, Murdoch D,** translators. Cambridge: Cambridge University Press; 1985.
15. **Damasio A.** Descartes' error: emotion, reason and the human brain. London: Vintage; 1999.
16. **Bhugra D.** Mental health for nations. Int Rev Psychiatry. 2016; **28**(4):342–74.
17. **Birchwood M, MacMillan F.** Early intervention in schizophrenia. Aust NZ J Psychiatry. 1993; **27**:374–8.
18. **Birchwood M, Fiorillo A.** The critical period for early intervention. Psychiatr Rehabil Skills. 2000; **4**:182–98.
19. **Insel TR.** The arrival of preemptive psychiatry. Early Interv Psychiatry. 2007; **1**:5–6.
20. **Stafford MR, Jackson H, Mayo-Wilson E, Morrison A, Kendall T.** Early interventions to prevent psychosis: systematic review and meta-analysis. BMJ. 2013; **346**:185.
21. **Tang JYM, Wong GHY, Hui CLM, Lam MML, Chiu CPY, Chan SKW,** et al. Early intervention for psychosis in Hong Kong—the EASY programme. Early Interv Psychiatry. 2010; **4**:214–19.
22. **Chen EYH, Tang JYM, Hui CLM, Chiu CPY, Lam MML, Law CW,** et al. Three-year outcome of phase-specific early intervention for first-episode psychosis: a cohort study in Hong Kong. Early Interv Psychiatry. 2011; **5**:315–23.
23. **Fowler D, Hodgekins J, Howells L, Millward M, Ivins A, Taylor G,** et al. Can targeted early intervention improve functional recovery in psychosis? A historical control evaluation of the effectiveness of different models of early intervention service provision in Norfolk 1998–2007. Early Interv Psychiatry. 2009; **3**:282–8.
24. **Craig T, Garety P, Power P, Rahaman N, Colbert S, Fornells-Ambrojo M,** et al. The Lambeth Early Onset (LEO) Team: randomised controlled trial of the effectiveness of specialised care for early psychosis. BMJ. 2004; **329**:1067.
25. **McGorry P, Killackey E, Yung A.** Early intervention in psychosis: concepts, evidence and future directions. World Psychiatry. 2008; **7**:148–56.
26. **Mizuno M, Suzuki M, Matsumoto K, Murakami M, Takeshi K, Miyakoshi T,** et al. Clinical practise and research activities for early psychiatric intervention at Japanese leading centres. Early Interv Psychiatry. 2009; **3**:5–9.
27. **Roberts N, Kitchiner N, Kenardy J, Bisson J.** Systematic review and meta-analysis of multiple-session early interventions following traumatic events. Am J Psychiatry. 2009; **166**:293–301.
28. **Adler A, Bliese P, McGurk D, Hoge CW, Castro CA.** Battlemind bebriefing and battlemind training as early interventions with soldiers returning from Iraq: randomization by platoon. J Psychol Clin Psychiatry. 2009; **77**:928–40.
29. **Chanen A, Jackson H, McCutcheon L, Jovev M, Dudgeon P, Yuen HP,** et al. Early intervention for adolescents with borderline personality disorder using cognitive analytic therapy: randomised controlled trial. Br J Psychiatry. 2008; **193**:477–84.
30. **LeGrange D, Loeb KL.** Early identification and treatment of eating disorders: prodrome to syndrome. Early Interv Psychiatry. 2007; **1**:27–39.

Chapter 4

Brain changes in the early course of schizophrenia

Matcheri S. Keshavan, Paulo Lizano, and Jaya Padmanabhan

Introduction

Schizophrenia and related psychotic disorders are common, and are among the most highly disabling illnesses in all of medicine. While the causes of psychotic disorders remain poorly understood, there have been remarkable advances in our understanding of its pathophysiology in recent years. 'Facts' of schizophrenia such as its adolescent onset, premorbid deficits, post-onset functional decline, and high heritability [1] suggest that studies of the early course of schizophrenia—in the premorbid, prodromal, and first episode—can help elucidate the etiopathogenesis of this illness. In this chapter, we review extant literature including our work in the *neurobiology* of early-course psychotic disorders using neurocognitive, structural, functional, and spectroscopic neuroimaging, as well as electrophysiological and sleep studies. Next, we will briefly review the models of *pathogenesis* that can help with understanding how the observed brain abnormalities might emerge. Finally, we review the *aetiology* of psychotic disorders and discuss the potential implications of these observations for their treatment and prevention.

What are the alterations in brain structure and function? Insights into neurobiology

Grey matter reductions

Brain structural alterations have been observed in schizophrenia since the beginning of the twentieth century, with early pneumo-encephalographic studies and post-mortem brain studies [2] showing enlarged cerebral ventricles and reduced brain parenchyma. Computed tomography (CT) scan studies in the

1970s confirmed these findings [3–7]. Magnetic resonance imaging (MRI) studies subsequently showed widespread grey matter (GM) reductions, notably in the heteromodal association cortex and limbic regions [8–13]. GM alterations appear to be present early in the illness [8, 14], progress during the first few years of the illness [15], may be related to the genetic susceptibility of this illness, and are present in the premorbid [16] and prodromal phases of the disorder [17, 18]. The GM alterations may predict poor outcome in first-episode patients [19, 20]. However, the precise nature of GM impairments, and their causes, remain unclear.

White matter alterations

Alterations in white matter (WM) tracts such as the corpus callosum, cingulum, arcuate, and the uncinate fasciculi [21] have been reported in schizophrenia. WM alterations such as corpus callosum reductions are present at illness onset [22] and are correlated with cognitive impairments [21]. Studies of WM connectivity have been made possible by diffusion tensor imaging (DTI) and fractional anisotropy (FA), the latter of which indexes the directional integrity of water diffusion along the axis of tissue elements, such as axons, and measures such diffusion from 0 (random diffusion) to 1 (unidirectional diffusion). Magnetic transfer spectroscopy has shown evidence of bioenergetic alterations in brains of patients with schizophrenia [23]. Free water imaging on DTI can be used to measure extracellular volume as a potential surrogate biomarker of neuroinflammation. Using this approach, Pasternak and colleagues [24] have reported a significant increase in the extracellular volume in both white and grey matter in early-course schizophrenia patients. Interestingly, WM alterations appear to be correlated with indices of brain elevations such as increased levels of interleukin-6 and C-reactive protein in early-course schizophrenia [25].

Alterations in brain function and connectivity

Functional imaging studies have produced robust evidence of altered brain function [26–30] consistent with the observed structural alterations early in the illness. In general, BOLD fMRI studies have demonstrated reduced task-related activity of prefrontal and temporal cortices (hypofrontality) in first-episode antipsychotic-naive schizophrenia patients [31]. Structural, DTI, and functional imaging studies, together, have pointed to widespread disturbances in brain connectivity in schizophrenia. DTI, as well as resting state fMRI studies, combined with recent techniques derived from graph theory, have shown a disruption of brain connectivity between central hub regions of the brain; this could lead to reduced communication capacity and altered functional brain dynamics seen in this illness [32].

Brain electrophysiology, electroencephalographic, event related potential, sleep studies

Electroencephalographic (EEG), event related potential (ERP), and eye-movement studies have cast considerable light on altered brain physiology in the early course of schizophrenia. First-episode schizophrenia patients show decreased amplitudes of P300 evoked potentials to oddball stimuli [33]. Eye-movement studies show increased antisaccade errors suggesting impairments in cognitive control [34]. There is also evidence of alterations in the steady-state gamma oscillations which appear to be correlated with impairments in working memory [35]. Pre-pulse inhibition, thought to reflect the process of sensory motor gating, is reduced in schizophrenia, and is also seen early in the illness [36]. Sleep EEG studies show evidence of reduced delta sleep [37] and spindle oscillations, which are thought to reflect memory consolidation processes [38].

Taken together, *in vivo* neuroimaging and electrophysiological studies strongly point to alterations in one or more neuronal elements in the schizophrenia brain. It is difficult, however, to draw conclusions about the nature of pathogenesis of this complex illness based on *in vivo* neurobiological studies alone. Neuropathological studies, longitudinal investigations, and studies of clinical and familial high-risk individuals have shed light on the questions of when and how the observed neurobiological alterations in schizophrenia may set in.

How might the brain changes emerge? Models of pathogenesis

Early and late developmental processes

Observations of premorbid cognitive and neuromotor deficits seen in the premorbid phase of schizophrenia [39] and the typical onset of psychotic symptoms around adolescence, point to the view that schizophrenia is a neurodevelopmental disorder. Some neuropathological studies implicate early neurodevelopmental migratory failure, mainly during the first and second trimesters of gestation, in the pathogenesis of schizophrenia. This view is based on observations of cortical neurons being more numerous in subcortical white matter brain regions in patients compared to controls, suggesting an impaired 'inside-out' migration of neuronal precursor cells from the subcortical to cortical regions [40]. Neuronal disarray in the hippocampal and anterior cingulate layer II also implicate early neurodevelopmental insults during neuronal migration [2, 41–44] (see Fig. 4.1)

Another, 'late' neurodevelopmental model posits neuropil reductions in schizophrenia resulting from an exaggeration of normative development pruning processes that happen around adolescence. Feinberg [45] initially suggested aberrant pruning of synapses (too much, too little, or the wrong synapses) around adolescence as the underlying pathogenesis of schizophrenia. Keshavan et al. [46] subsequently suggested an exaggerated pruning of synapses in this illness. While this has been supported by observations of decreased density of synapses in post-mortem brains of schizophrenia patients [47], the precise mechanisms have remained unclear. Adolescent neurodevelopment normally involves neuronal apoptosis ('programmed' cell death) and synaptic pruning [46]. Glutamate, via N-methyl D-aspartate (NMDA) activity, may be important for these neurodevelopmental processes of synaptic refinements and plasticity [48, 49]. NMDA receptor hypofunction has also been posited to account for a host of alterations such as disinhibition of meso-cortical dopaminergic tone, and for negative symptoms and cognitive deficits, by causing prefrontal cortical dysfunction, and has become one of the commonly accepted models of schizophrenia [48, 49]. Progressive GM reductions in clinically at-risk individuals

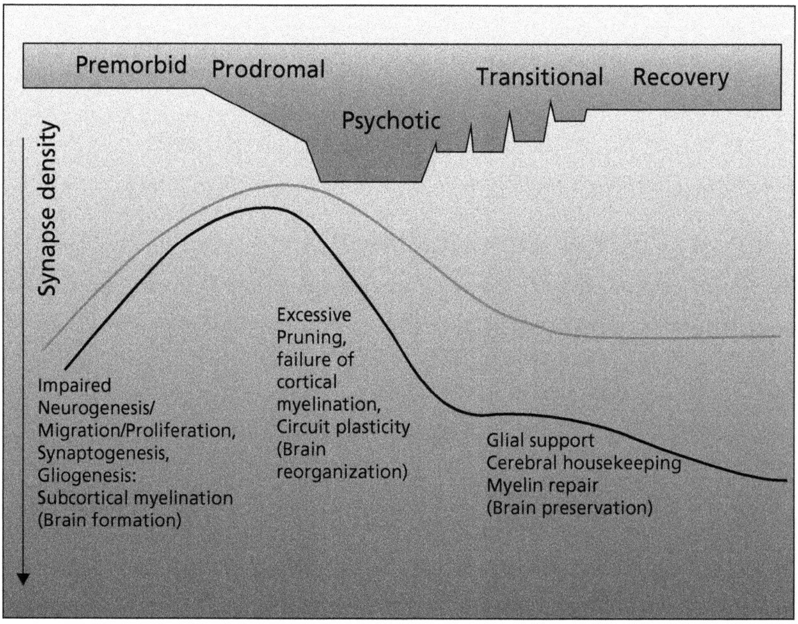

Fig. 4.1 Evolution of schizophrenia is linked to brain developmental processes.

who later convert to schizophrenia [50], 31P magnetic resonance spectroscopy (MRS) studies in first-episode schizophrenia showing impaired prefrontal membrane phospholipid metabolism, and proton MRS studies showing deficits in N-Acetyl aspartate (a marker of neuronal viability) [51–53] are all consistent with this possibility.

Neurochemical processes

NMDA receptor alterations can cause disinhibition of glutamatergic release [54] to layer III cells [55] causing excitotoxic damage. Indeed, a recent meta-analysis has shown increased levels of glutamate in MRS studies [56]. Glutamatergic abnormalities might be related to altered GABAergic function, for which there is increasing evidence [57]. Corticofugal glutamatergic neurons [55] reciprocally regulate mesocortical and mesolimbic dopaminergic transmission; such regulation may be altered in schizophrenia [58–62], leading to increased dopaminergic transmission in the mesolimbic pathway. This may account for positive symptoms, including paranoia, while hypodopaminergic mesocortical transmission may cause cognitive deficits and negative symptoms including avolition, anhedonia, and apathy [63, 64]. Recent positron emission tomography (PET) imaging studies in early-course schizophrenia and at-risk populations indeed show evidence of increased presynaptic dopamine neurotransmission in the ventral striatum [65].

Inflammatory, vascular, and oxidative stress mechanisms

Several other pathogenic mechanisms have been implicated in schizophrenia. A growing body of literature points to immune, inflammatory, oxidative stress, and microvascular processes. Large population-based studies of interleukin-6 (IL-6) and C-reactive protein (CRP) levels in healthy children and adolescents have shown an association with subsequent risk for schizophrenia [66, 67]. Studies of individuals at high risk for psychosis are beginning to support the inflammatory, oxidative stress, microvascular, and hypothalamic-pituitary axis hypothesis with the potential to predict conversion to psychosis [68–70]. Additional evidence from meta-analyses of first-episode, acutely relapsed, and schizophrenia patients has demonstrated significant changes in lymphocyte populations, cytokine expression, and oxidative stress, and some of these markers are affected by antipsychotic treatment [71–73]. To date, there are a growing number of studies investigating the role of these mechanisms on brain structure and function.

In schizophrenia, hippocampal volume reductions have been associated with a functional genetic polymorphism for IL-6, as well as peripheral reductions in brain-derived neurotrophic factor (BDNF) and increased levels of

IL-6 and cortisol [74–76]. Frontal grey matter volume reductions have been associated with a functional genetic polymorphism for IL-1β and increased peripheral vascular endothelial growth factor (VEGF) levels in individuals with schizophrenia [77, 78]. Also, BDNF met-allele carriers have smaller temporal and occipital grey matter volumes [79]. Interestingly, a study by Fillman et al. [80] showed that a schizophrenia subgroup with elevated peripheral inflammatory cytokines (IL-1β, IL-2, IL-8, and IL-18) showed a significant left pars opercularis volume reduction compared to the low inflammatory group [80].

Additionally, a longitudinal study of clinical high risk for psychosis subjects showed that the rate of prefrontal cortical thinning was significantly associated with higher levels of pro-inflammatory (TNFα, IL-2, and IFNθ) markers, and this effect was significantly greater among converters versus non-converters or control subjects [50]. Peripheral IL-6 and CRP levels have been associated with impaired anisotropy in schizophrenia [25]. Functionally, the IL-1β functional polymorphism has been associated with differential brain activation of the dorsolateral prefrontal cortex [81], while a PET imaging study of regional cerebral blood flow showed that the BDNF polymorphism is associated with differential hippocampal function [82]. PET studies suggest increases in activated microglia, though this literature is inconsistent. Another view that is gaining ground is that pathological angiogenic processes may be involved, with elevations of anti-angiogenic factors such as sFLT-1 in familial high-risk individuals, resulting in worsening symptomatology and progressive cortical thickness loss over time [70]. The interaction between immune, inflammatory, and angiogenic processes may contribute to a metabolic imbalance, leading to increased oxidative stress and, hence, neuronal damage. Together, all of these processes could lead to a failure of brain plasticity [83] and an imbalance between the excitatory and inhibitory neural processes, leading to the phenotypic manifestations of what we call schizophrenia.

Alterations in brain plasticity

Impaired mechanisms of cortical plasticity are also drawing increasing interest for their possible role in the pathophysiology of schizophrenia [83]. Plasticity may be subdivided into non-synaptic and synaptic plasticity. Non-synaptic plasticity encompasses processes that alter the intrinsic excitability of neurons through changes in the cell bodies, axons, or dendrites of neurons. Synaptic plasticity involves changes in the strength of synapses in response to changes in their activity, and includes long-term potentiation (an enhancement of the efficacy of synaptic transmission) and long-term depression (a decrease in the efficacy of synaptic transmission) [84, 85].

Several lines of evidence imply the existence of impaired cortical plasticity in schizophrenia. The observation that NMDA receptor antagonists, such as phencyclidine, can induce psychotic symptoms and cognitive impairment in healthy individuals led to the development of glutamatergic, NMDA receptor-based theories of schizophrenia [86]. If validated, these glutamatergic theories would indicate the existence of cortical plasticity deficits in schizophrenia. Long-term potentiation (LTP) in the hippocampus requires proper NMDA receptor and AMPA receptor function [87]; thus, abnormalities in NMDA receptor function (or associated processes) could concurrently lead to impaired cortical plasticity, cognitive impairment, and psychosis.

Additionally, electrophysiological protocols involving repetitive auditory stimuli have been used to demonstrate reduced habituation to repetitive stimuli in psychosis, potentially implying reduced plasticity. For example, children with psychosis and those at high risk of psychosis demonstrated reduced change in the amplitude of the auditory N100 (an obligatory response generated in the auditory cortex after a sound) during a sequence of repetitive auditory stimuli [88]. Mismatch negativity—the brain's electrophysiological response to a deviant stimulus within a train of repetitive stimuli—has been shown to be consistently abnormal in schizophrenia [89]. This abnormality may reflect impairments in NMDA receptor-mediated processes, as it can also be induced in healthy subjects by administering NMDA receptor antagonists [90].

Non-invasive brain stimulation, including transcranial magnetic stimulation (TMS) and transcranial electrical stimulation (tES), offers the opportunity to probe mechanisms of both LTP-like plasticity and long-term depression-like (LTD-like) plasticity. (The terms 'LTP-like' and 'LTD-like' are used to describe plasticity induced by non-invasive brain stimulation studies, since LTP and LTD cannot be confirmed, on the cellular level, in living humans.) TMS stimulates brain regions by using magnetic pulses to induce brief electrical currents, while tES directly applies weak electrical currents to the head. Depending on protocol parameters, repetitive TMS or tES can be excitatory, causing LTP-like plasticity, or inhibitory, causing LTD-like plasticity [91, 92]. Changes in amplitudes of motor-evoked potentials following an excitatory or inhibitory protocol can be used to quantify LTP-like and LTD-like plasticity, respectively. Multiple studies using repetitive TMS or tES have found evidence of both impaired LTP-like and LTD-like plasticity in schizophrenia (reviewed in Bhandari et al. [93]). However, these studies have focused on the motor cortex, as the measurement of cortical plasticity outside the motor cortex is less established.

Further research is needed to determine whether cortical plasticity is more impaired in particular brain regions, such as the prefrontal cortex, and whether impaired plasticity accounts for cognitive impairment or symptom severity.

With respect to early-course psychosis, future research may help elucidate whether measures of cortical plasticity steadily decline in this period, along with structural and functional brain measures.

Post-illness onset pathogenic processes

Grey and white matter reductions in schizophrenia may also result from processes other than the pathophysiological substrate of the illness. Schizophrenia is associated with high rates of alcohol and nicotine use disorders, both of which may have the consequence of brain structural alterations [94, 95]. Cannabis may also increase grey matter volume loss [96]. Antipsychotics may contribute to GM and WM loss [97, 98]. The processes of age-related cognitive decline and brain change may also be amplified in schizophrenia [99]. Psychosocial impoverishment, which characterizes many patients with prominent negative symptoms and institutionalization, may also contribute to brain volume loss secondary to disuse atrophy as is seen in neuromuscular disorders [100].

Why do neurobiological alterations occur? Genetic, environmental, and epigenetic aetiology

Family, adoptive, and twin studies have firmly established genetic factors as among the strongest aetiological factors in schizophrenia. Schizophrenia has high (approximately 70–80 per cent) heritability. However, a large portion of this heritability remains unclear, though substantive advances have been in recent years due to the advent of genome-wide association (GWAS) studies. A recent large-scale GWAS study [101] showed 108 schizophrenia-associated genetic loci involving 341 protein-coding genes, which reached genome-wide significance. Among these genetic loci were genes related to previously implicated theories of schizophrenia pathophysiology; that is, several glutamatergic genes and one dopaminergic gene (DRD2). One particular series of observations has garnered a great deal of attention, and helps 'connect the dots' among several clinical and scientific observations. Previous GWAS studies had shown that a region of DNA located on chromosome 6, comprising the major histocompatibility (MHC) region, was strongly associated with schizophrenia risk. However, the precise genes and the molecular mechanisms underlying this genetic locus had remained elusive until recently. An exciting observation at Harvard, by Stephan and colleagues, rekindled interest in the synaptic hyper-pruning hypothesis [102]. Complement proteins, which are known components of the immune system, are repurposed for another role (i.e. tagging synapses for phagocytosis), and hence, in synaptic pruning processes during adolescence.

Finally, a recent study [103] showed, again using the large-scale GWAS data, that genes involved in the complement cascade—notably (complement)C4A and C4B—are part of this gene location, and alleles with the highest C4A expression were among the most strongly associated with schizophrenia. They also showed that C4A (messenger)mRNA levels were higher in the brains of schizophrenia patients than control brains; further, mice bred for higher C4 activity showed increased synaptic pruning during brain development (see Fig. 4.2).

Another interesting line of work that may shed some light on aberrant neurodevelopment processes involves the role of perineuronal nets (PNNs). PNNs are extracellular matrix proteins that form a lattice-like scaffolding around soma, axons, and dendrites, and are involved in regulation of synapse formation, functioning, and refinements. They develop postnatally, reaching their maximum around adolescence. An improper development of PNNs could conceivably underlie aberrant synapse pruning processes; indeed, recent post-mortem studies support this possibility (for a review, see Bitanihirwe et al. [104]). PNNs are regulated by genes such as metalloproteases, that have been implicated in recent GWAS studies [101]. Taken together, these tantalizing observations point to the possibility of identifying subgroups of psychotic

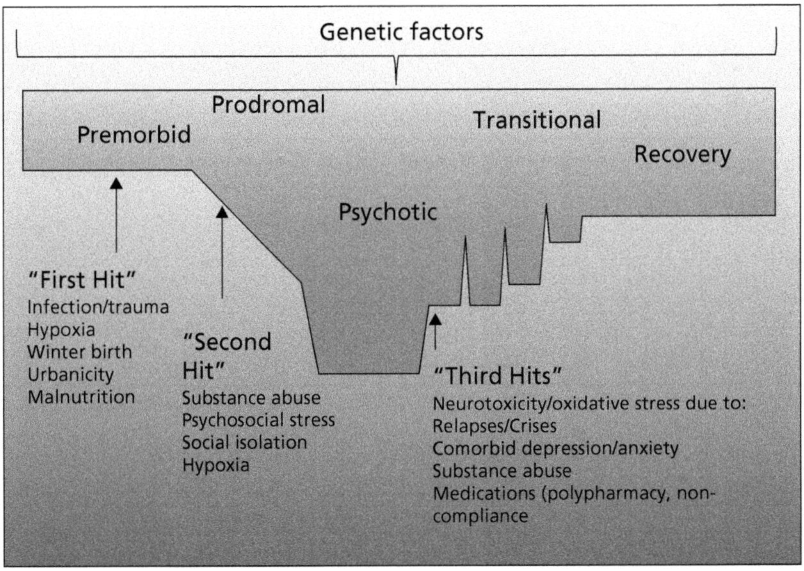

Fig. 4.2 Schizophrenia may be linked to sequential pathophysiological hits early in development, around adolescence, and after illness onset.

disorders where a known set of risk genes work, via a known pathophysiological mechanism, to produce an observable illness phenotype.

A continuing challenge in understanding psychotic disorders is that many biological findings and the implicated susceptibility genes overlap not only between psychotic disorders, but also between psychotic, affective, and developmental disorders [105]. For this reason, research domain criteria (R-DoC) approaches, recently outlined by Insel and colleagues [106], are important to advance the field by examining data across multiple disorders, and also to capture the continuous variation between health and disease. Recent studies such as the Bipolar and Schizophrenia Network for Intermediate Phenotypes (B-SNIP) are beginning to show that it is possible to identify biological subtypes that cut across DSM (Diagnostic and Statistical Manual) psychotic disorders, and may show better validation by external validators such as neuroimaging data [107].

What are the therapeutic implications?

The pharmacological treatment of schizophrenia is in need of a paradigm shift. Following the introduction of antipsychotics into clinical practice over half a century ago, progress has been modest. Current treatments are fairly effective in treating some aspects of the illness, but not others. Presently, we lack proven preventative strategies or effective treatments for the prodromal phase when substantial damage occurs. Persons with schizophrenia demonstrate extremely varied responses to the different therapeutic interventions, and our lack of reliable methods to predict such variations necessitates a trial-and-error treatment strategy. Treatments continue to be associated with significant adverse effects. In large measure, this state of affairs is the result of an inadequate understanding of the pathophysiological substrate underlying this complex syndrome. While much effort has gone into modifying and changing existing antidopaminergic medications, the added benefits of such incremental research have been limited.

Spectacular recent advances in genetics and molecular neurobiology, however, generate enthusiasm about the potential of applying these strategies to substantially upgrade the drug treatment of schizophrenia. Genomic advances now enable a more precise dissection of the heterogeneity of schizophrenia and the development of therapeutic agents directed at defined 'disease-specific' targets. Such advances will allow the schizophrenia syndrome to be deconstructed into aetiologically distinct subgroups. There is likely to be more dividend from systematic investigation of non-dopaminergic mechanisms that may underlie schizophrenia pathophysiology. Future research needs to invest in clinically meaningful and translationally relevant animal models and *in vivo* screening methods for novel therapeutic targets and optimal clinical trial design. As we wait for these methodologies to deliver on their promise in the near future, however, it is important to more optimally utilize existing agents by practicing evidence-based and measurement-based medicine.

References

1. **Tandon R, Keshavan MS, Nasrallah HA.** Schizophrenia, 'Just the facts': what we know in 2008. Part 1: overview. Schizophr Res. 2008 Mar; **100**(1–3):4–19.
2. **Harrison PJ.** The neuropathology of schizophrenia. A critical review of the data and their interpretation. Brain. 1999; **122**(Pt 4):593–624.
3. **Johnstone EC, Crow TJ, Frith CD, Husband J, Kreel L.** Cerebral ventricular size and cognitive impairment in chronic schizophrenia. Lancet. 1976; **2**(7992):924–6.
4. **Johnstone EC, Crow TJ, Frith CD, Stevens M, Kreel L, Husband J.** The dementia of dementia praecox. Acta Psychiatr Scand. 1978; **57**(4):305–24.
5. **Reveley AM, Reveley MA, Clifford CA, Murray RM.** Cerebral ventricular size in twins discordant for schizophrenia. Lancet. 1982; **1**(8271):540–1.
6. **Reveley AM, Reveley MA, Murray RM.** Enlargement of cerebral ventricles in schizophrenics is confined to those without known genetic predisposition. Lancet. 1983; **2**(8348):525. doi:S0140-6736(83)90562-7 [pii]
7. **Reveley AM, Reveley MA, Murray RM.** Cerebral ventricular enlargement in non-genetic schizophrenia: a controlled twin study. Br J Psychiatry. 1984; **144**:89–93.
8. **Ellison-Wright I, Glahn DC, Laird AR, Thelen SM, Bullmore E.** The anatomy of first-episode and chronic schizophrenia: an anatomical likelihood estimation meta-analysis. Am J Psychiatry. 2008; **165**(8):1015–23. doi:10.1176/appi.ajp.2008.07101562
9. **Honea R, Crow TJ, Passingham D, Mackay CE.** Regional deficits in brain volume in schizophrenia: a meta-analysis of voxel-based morphometry studies. Am J Psychiatry. 2005; **162**(12):2233–45. doi:162/12/2233 [pii] 0.1176/appi.ajp.162.12.2233
10. **Shenton ME, Dickey CC, Frumin M, McCarley RW.** A review of MRI findings in schizophrenia. Schizophr Res. 2001; **49**(1–2):1–52.
11. **Wright IC, Ellison ZR, Sharma T, Friston KJ, Murray RM, McGuire PK.** Mapping of grey matter changes in schizophrenia. Schizophr Res. 1999; **35**(1):1–14. doi:S0920-9964(98)00094-2 [pii]
12. **Wright IC, Rabe-Hesketh S, Woodruff PW, David AS, Murray RM, Bullmore ET.** Meta-analysis of regional brain volumes in schizophrenia. Am J Psychiatry. 2000; **157**(1):16–25.
13. **Wright IC, Sharma T, Ellison ZR, McGuire PK, Friston KJ, Brammer MJ**, et al. Supra-regional brain systems and the neuropathology of schizophrenia. Cereb Cortex. 1999; **9**(4):366–78.
14. **Meda SA, Giuliani NR, Calhoun VD, Jagannathan K, Schretlen DJ, Pulver A**, et al. A large scale (N=400) investigation of gray matter differences in schizophrenia using optimized voxel-based morphometry. Schizophr Res. 2008; **101**(1–3):95–105.
15. **Farrow TF, Whitford TJ, Williams LM, Gomes L, Harris AW.** Diagnosis-related regional gray matter loss over two years in first episode schizophrenia and bipolar disorder. Biol Psychiatry. 2005; **58**(9):713–23.

16. **Keshavan MS, Diwadkar VA, Montrose DM, Rajarethinam R, Sweeney JA.** Premorbid indicators and risk for schizophrenia: a selective review and update. Schizophr Res. 2005; **79**(1):45–57. doi:S0920-9964(05)00295-1 [pii] 10.1016/j.schres.2005.07.004
17. **Keshavan MS, Diwadkar V, Rosenberg DR.** Developmental biomarkers in schizophrenia and other psychiatric disorders: common origins, different trajectories? Epidemiol Psichiatr Soc. 2005; **14**(4):188–93.
18. **Pantelis C, Velakoulis D, McGorry PD, Wood SJ, Suckling J, Phillips LJ,** et al. Neuroanatomical abnormalities before and after onset of psychosis: a cross-sectional and longitudinal MRI comparison. Lancet. 2003; **361**(9354):281–8. doi:10.1016/S0140-6736(03)12323-9
19. **Mitelman SA, Brickman AM, Shihabuddin L, Newmark RE, Hazlett EA, Haznedar MM,** et al. A comprehensive assessment of gray and white matter volumes and their relationship to outcome and severity in schizophrenia. Neuroimage. 2007; **37**(2): 449–62. doi:S1053-8119(07)00403-X [pii] 10.1016/j.neuroimage.2007.04.070
20. **Prasad KM, Sahni SD, Rohm BR, Keshavan MS.** Dorsolateral prefrontal cortex morphology and short-term outcome in first-episode schizophrenia. Psychiatry Res. 2005; **140**(2):147–55. doi:S0925-4927(05)00113-7 [pii] 10.1016/j.pscychresns.2004.05.009
21. **Kubicki M, McCarley R, Westin CF, Park HJ, Maier S, Kikinis R,** et al. A review of diffusion tensor imaging studies in schizophrenia. J Psychiatr Res. 2007; **41**(1–2):15–30.
22. **Keshavan MS, Diwadkar VA, Harenski K, Rosenberg DR, Sweeney JA, Pettegrew JW.** Abnormalities of the corpus callosum in first episode, treatment naive schizophrenia. J Neurol Neurosurg Psychiatry. 2002; **72**(6):757–60.
23. **Du F, Cooper AJ, Thida T, Sehovic S, Lukas SE, Cohen BM,** et al. In vivo evidence for cerebral bioenergetic abnormalities in schizophrenia measured using 31P magnetization transfer spectroscopy. JAMA Psychiatry. 2014 Jan; **71**(1):19–27.
24. **Pasternak O, Westin CF, Bouix S, Seidman LJ, Goldstein JM, Woo TU,** et al. Excessive extracellular volume reveals a neurodegenerative pattern in schizophrenia onset. J Neurosci. 2012 Nov 28; **32**(48):17365–72.
25. **Prasad KM, Upton CH, Nimgaonkar VL, Keshavan MS.** Differential susceptibility of white matter tracts to inflammatory mediators in schizophrenia: an integrated DTI study. Schizophr Res. 2015 Jan; **161**(1):119–25.
26. **Buckholtz JW, Meyer-Lindenberg A, Honea RA, Straub RE, Pezawas L, Egan MF,** et al. Allelic variation in RGS4 impacts functional and structural connectivity in the human brain. J Neurosci. 2007; **27**(7):1584–93. doi:27/7/1584 [pii] 10.1523/JNEUROSCI.5112-06.2007
27. **Kindermann SS, Karimi A, Symonds L, Brown GG, Jeste DV.** Review of functional magnetic resonance imaging in schizophrenia. Schizophr Res. 1997; **27**(2–3):143–56. doi:S0920-9964(97)00063-7 [pii] 10.1016/S0920-9964(97)00063-7
28. **Lv YT, Yang H, Wang DY, Li SY, Han Y, Zhu CZ,** et al. Correlations in spontaneous activity and gray matter density between left and right sensoriomotor areas of pianists. Neuroreport. 2008; **19**(6):631–4. doi:10.1097/WNR.0b013e3282fa6da0 00001756-200804160-00006 [pii]
29. **Park HJ, Lee JD, Chun JW, Seok JH, Yun M, Oh MK,** et al. Cortical surface-based analysis of 18F-FDG PET: measured metabolic abnormalities in schizophrenia are affected by cortical structural abnormalities. Neuroimage. 2006; **31**(4):1434–44. doi:S1053-8119(06)00100-5 [pii] 10.1016/j.neuroimage.2006.02.001

30. **Zakzanis KK, Poulin P, Hansen KT, Jolic D.** Searching the schizophrenic brain for temporal lobe deficits: a systematic review and meta-analysis. Psychol Med. 2000; **30**(3):491–504.

31. **Gong Q, Lui S, Sweeney JA.** A selective review of cerebral abnormalities in patients with first-episode schizophrenia before and after treatment. Am J Psychiatry. 2016 Mar 1; **173**(3):232–43.

32. **van den Heuvel MP, Sporns O, Collin G, Scheewe T, Mandl RC, Cahn W,** et al. Abnormal rich club organization and functional brain dynamics in schizophrenia. JAMA Psychiatry. 2013 Aug; **70**(8):783–92.

33. **Ford JM.** Schizophrenia: the broken P300 and beyond. Psychophysiology. 1999; **36**:667–82.

34. **Reilly JL, Harris MSH, Keshavan MS, Sweeney JA.** Abnormalities in visually guided saccades suggest corticofugal dysregulation in never-treated schizophrenia. Biol Psychiatry. 2005; **57**(2):145–54.

35. **Spencer KM, Nestor PG, Perlmutter R, Niznikiewicz MA, Klump MC, Frumin M,** et al. Neural synchrony indexes, disordered perception and cognition in schizophrenia. Proc Natl Acad Sci U S A. 2004; **101**:17288–93.

36. **Braff DL, Light GA.** The use of neurophysiological endophenotypes to understand the genetic basis of schizophrenia. Dialogues Clin Neurosci. 2005; **7**(2):125–35.

37. **Keshavan MS, Reynolds CF 3rd, Miewald MJ, Montrose DM, Sweeney JA, Vasko RC Jr,** et al. Delta sleep deficits in schizophrenia: evidence from automated analyses of sleep data. Arch Gen Psychiatry. 1998; **55**(5):443–8.

38. **Manoach DS, Demanuele C, Wamsley EJ, Vangel M, Montrose DM, Miewald J,** et al. Sleep spindle deficits in antipsychotic-naïve early course schizophrenia and in non-psychotic first-degree relatives. Front Hum Neurosci. 2014 Oct 7; **8**:762.

39. **Keshavan MS, Diwadkar VA, Montrose DM, Rajarethinam R, Sweeney JA.** Premorbid indicators and risk for schizophrenia: a selective review and update. Schizophr Res. 2005; **79**(1):45–57.

40. **Arnold SE.** Neurodevelopmental abnormalities in schizophrenia: insights from neuropathology. Developmental Psychopathology. 1999; **11**(3):439–56.

41. **Conrad AJ, Abebe T, Austin R, Forsythe S, Scheibel AB.** Hippocampal pyramidal cell disarray in schizophrenia as a bilateral phenomenon. Arch Gen Psychiatry. 1991; **48**(5): 413–17.

42. **Conrad AJ, Scheibel AB.** Schizophrenia and the hippocampus: the embryological hypothesis extended. Schizophr Bull. 1987; **13**(4):577–87.

43. **Jonsson SA, Luts A, Guldberg-Kjaer N, Brun A.** Hippocampal pyramidal cell disarray correlates negatively to cell number: implications for the pathogenesis of schizophrenia. Eur Arch Psychiatry Clin Neurosci. 1997; **247**(3): 120–7.

44. **Kovelman JA, Scheibel AB.** A neurohistological correlate of schizophrenia. Biol Psychiatry. 1984; **19**(12):1601–21.

45. **Feinberg I.** Schizophrenia: caused by a fault in programmed synaptic elimination during adolescence? J Psychiatr Res. 1982–3; **17**(4):319–34.

46. **Keshavan MS, Anderson S, Pettegrew JW.** Is schizophrenia due to excessive synaptic pruning in the prefrontal cortex? The Feinberg hypothesis revisited. J Psychiatr Res. 1994; **28**(3):239–65.

47. **Glantz LA, Lewis DA.** Decreased dendritic spine density on prefrontal cortical pyramidal neurons in schizophrenia. Arch Gen Psychiatry. 2000 Jan; **57**(1):65–73.

48. **Goff DC, Coyle JT.** The emerging role of glutamate in the pathophysiology and treatment of schizophrenia. Am J Psychiatry. 2001; **158**(9):1367–77.
49. **Lindsley CW, Shipe WD, Wolkenberg SE, Theberge CR, Williams DL** Jr, **Sur C, Kinney GG.** Progress towards validating the NMDA receptor hypofunction hypothesis of schizophrenia. Curr Top Med Chem. 2006; **6**(8):771–85.
50. **Cannon TD, Chung Y, He G, Sun D, Jacobson A, van Erp TG,** et al. Progressive reduction in cortical thickness as psychosis develops: a multisite longitudinal neuroimaging study of youth at elevated clinical risk. Biol Psychiatry. 2015 Jan 15; 77(2):147–57.
51. **Keshavan MS, Sanders RD, Pettegrew JW, Dombrowsky SM, Panchalingam KS.** Frontal lobe metabolism and cerebral morphology in schizophrenia: 31P MRS and MRI studies. Schizophr Res. 1993; **10**(3): 241–6.
52. **Keshavan MS, Stanley JA, Montrose DM, Minshew NJ, Pettegrew JW.** Prefrontal membrane phospholipid metabolism of child and adolescent offspring at risk for schizophrenia or schizoaffective disorder: an in vivo 31P MRS study. Mol Psychiatry. 2003; **8**(3):316–23, 251. doi:10.1038/sj.mp.4001325 4001325 [pii]
53. **Keshavan MS, Stanley JA, Pettegrew JW.** Magnetic resonance spectroscopy in schizophrenia: methodological issues and findings—part II. Biol Psychiatry. 2000; **48**(5):369–80. doi:S0006-3223(00)00940-9 [pii]
54. **Deutsch SI, Rosse RB, Schwartz BL, Mastropaolo J.** A revised excitotoxic hypothesis of schizophrenia: therapeutic implications. Clin Neuropharmacol. 2001; **24**(1):43–9.
55. **Lewis DA, Glantz LA, Pierri JN, Sweet RA.** Altered cortical glutamate neurotransmission in schizophrenia: evidence from morphological studies of pyramidal neurons. Ann N Y Acad Sci. 2003; **1003**:102–12.
56. **Merritt K, Egerton A, Kempton MJ, Taylor MJ, McGuire PK.** Nature of glutamate alterations in schizophrenia: a meta-analysis of proton magnetic resonance spectroscopy studies. JAMA Psychiatry. 2016 Jul 1; **73**(7):665–74.
57. **Benes FM, Berretta S.** Amygdalo-entorhinal inputs to the hippocampal formation in relation to schizophrenia. Ann N Y Acad Sci. 2000; **911**:293–304.
58. **Del Arco A, Mora F.** Neurotransmitters and prefrontal cortex-limbic system interactions: implications for plasticity and psychiatric disorders. J Neural Transm. 2009; **116**(8):941–52. doi:10.1007/s00702-009-0243-8
59. **Seeman P.** Glutamate and dopamine components in schizophrenia. J Psychiatry Neurosci. 2009; **34**(2):143–9.
60. **Seeman P, Guan HC.** Glutamate agonists for treating schizophrenia have affinity for dopamine D2High and D3 receptors. Synapse. 2009; **63**(8):705–9. doi:10.1002/syn.20673
61. **Tanaka S.** Dopaminergic control of working memory and its relevance to schizophrenia: a circuit dynamics perspective. Neuroscience. 2006; **139**(1):153–71. doi:S0306-4522(05)00972-3 [pii] 10.1016/j.neuroscience.2005.08.070
62. **Winterer G, Weinberger DR.** Genes, dopamine and cortical signal-to-noise ratio in schizophrenia. Trends Neurosci. 2004; **27**(11):683–90. doi:S0166-2236(04)00259-0 [pii] 10.1016/j.tins.2004.08.002
63. **Deutch AY.** The regulation of subcortical dopamine systems by the prefrontal cortex: interactions of central dopamine systems and the pathogenesis of schizophrenia. J Neural Transm Suppl. 1992; **36**:61–89.

64. **Kapur S.** Psychosis as a state of aberrant salience: a framework linking biology, phenomenology, and pharmacology in schizophrenia. Am J Psychiatry. 2003; **160**(1):13–23.
65. **Howes O, McCutcheon R, Stone J.** Glutamate and dopamine in schizophrenia: an update for the 21st century. J Psychopharmacol. 2015 Feb; **29**(2):97–115.
66. **Khandaker GM, Pearson RM, Zammit S, Lewis G, Jones PB.** Association of serum interleukin 6 and C-reactive protein in childhood with depression and psychosis in young adult life: a population-based longitudinal study. JAMA Psychiatry. 2014; **71**(10):1121–8. doi: 10.1001/jamapsychiatry.2014.1332
67. **Metcalf SA, Jones PB, Nordstrom T, Timonen M, Mäki P, Miettunen J,** et al. Serum C-reactive protein in adolescence and risk of schizophrenia in adulthood: a prospective birth cohort study. Brain Behav Immun. 2017 Jan; **59**:253–9. doi: 10.1016/j.bbi.2016.09.008.
68. **Perkins DO, Jeffries CD, Addington J, Bearden CE, Cadenhead KS, Cannon TD,** et al. Towards a psychosis risk blood diagnostic for persons experiencing high-risk symptoms: preliminary results from the NAPLS project. Schizophrenia Bull. 2015; **41**(2):419–28.
69. **Hayes LN, Severance EG, Leek JT, Gressitt KL, Rohleder C, Coughlin JM,** et al. Inflammatory molecular signature associated with infectious agents in psychosis. Schizophrenia Bull. 2014; **40**(5):963–72.
70. **Lizano PL, Keshavan MS, Tandon N, Mathew IT, Mothi SS, Montrose DM,** et al. Angiogenic and immune signatures in plasma of young relatives at familial high-risk for psychosis and first-episode patients: A preliminary study. Schizophrenia Res. 2016; **170**(1):115–22.
71. **Miller BJ, Gassama B, Sebastian D, Buckley P, Mellor A.** Meta-analysis of lymphocytes in schizophrenia: clinical status and antipsychotic effects. Biol Psychiatry. 2013; **73**(10):993–9.
72. **Miller BJ, Buckley P, Seabolt W, Mellor A, Kirkpatrick B.** Meta-analysis of cytokine alterations in schizophrenia: clinical status and antipsychotic effects. Biol Psychiatry. 2011; **70**(7):663–71.
73. **Flatow J, Buckley P, Miller BJ.** Meta-analysis of oxidative stress in schizophrenia. Biol Psychiatry. 2013; **74**(6):400–9.
74. **Kalmady SV, Venkatasubramanian G, Shivakumar V, Gautham S, Subramaniam A, Jose DA,** et al. Relationship between Interleukin-6 gene polymorphism and hippocampal volume in antipsychotic-naive schizophrenia: evidence for differential susceptibility? PloS One. 2014; **9**(5):e96021.
75. **Mondelli V, Cattaneo A, Belvederi Murri M, Di Forti M, Handley R, Hepgul N,** et al. Stress and inflammation reduce brain-derived neurotrophic factor expression in first-episode psychosis: a pathway to smaller hippocampal volume. J Clin Psychiatry. 2011; **72**(12):1677–84.
76. **Mondelli V, Pariante CM, Navari S, Aas M, D'Albenzio A, Di Forti M,** et al. Higher cortisol levels are associated with smaller left hippocampal volume in first-episode psychosis. Schizophrenia Res. 2010; **119**(1–3):75–8.
77. **Meisenzahl EM, Rujescu D, Kirner A, Giegling I, Kathmann N, Leinsinger G,** et al. Association of an interleukin-1beta genetic polymorphism with altered brain structure in patients with schizophrenia. Am J Psychiatry. 2001; **158**(8):1316–9.

78. **Pillai A, Howell KR, Ahmed AO, Weinberg D, Allen KM, Bruggemann J**, et al. Association of serum VEGF levels with prefrontal cortex volume in schizophrenia. Mol Psychiatry. 2016; **21**(5):686–92.
79. **Ho BC, Milev P, O'Leary DS, Librant A, Andreasen NC, Wassink TH.** Cognitive and magnetic resonance imaging brain morphometric correlates of brain-derived neurotrophic factor Val66Met gene polymorphism in patients with schizophrenia and healthy volunteers. Archiv Gen Psychiatry. 2006; **63**(7):731–40.
80. **Fillman SG, Weickert TW, Lenroot RK, Catts SV, Bruggemann JM, Catts VS**, et al. Elevated peripheral cytokines characterize a subgroup of people with schizophrenia displaying poor verbal fluency and reduced Broca's area volume. Mol Psychiatry. 2016; **21**(8):1090–8.
81. **Fatjo-Vilas M, Pomarol-Clotet E, Salvador R, Monte GC, Gomar JJ, Sarro S**, et al. Effect of the interleukin-1beta gene on dorsolateral prefrontal cortex function in schizophrenia: a genetic neuroimaging study. Biol Psychiatry. 2012; **72**(9):758–65.
82. **Eisenberg DP, Ianni AM, Wei SM, Kohn PD, Kolachana B, Apud J**, et al. Brain-derived neurotrophic factor (BDNF) Val(66)Met polymorphism differentially predicts hippocampal function in medication-free patients with schizophrenia. Mol Psychiatry. 2013; **18**(6):713–20.
83. **Keshavan MS, Mehta UM, Padmanabhan JL, Shah JL.** Dysplasticity, metaplasticity, and schizophrenia: implications for risk, illness, and novel interventions. Dev Psychopathol. 2015; **27**(2):615–35. doi:10.1017/S095457941500019X
84. **Bliss TV, Collingridge GL.** A synaptic model of memory: long-term potentiation in the hippocampus. Nature. 1993; **361**(6407):31–9. doi:10.1038/361031a0
85. **Lomo T.** The discovery of long-term potentiation. Philos Trans R Soc Lond B Biol Sci. 2003; **358**(1432):617–20. doi:10.1098/rstb.2002.1226
86. **Javitt DC, Zukin SR.** Recent advances in the phencyclidine model of schizophrenia. Am J Psychiatry. 1991; **148**(10):1301–8.
87. **Morris RG, Anderson E, Lynch GS, Baudry M.** Selective impairment of learning and blockade of long-term potentiation by an N-methyl-D-aspartate receptor antagonist, AP5. Nature. 1986; **319**(6056):774–6. doi:10.1038/319774a0
88. **Gonzalez-Heydrich J, Enlow MB, D'Angelo E, Seidman LJ, Gumlak S, Kim A**, et al. N100 repetition suppression indexes neuroplastic defects in clinical high risk and psychotic youth. Neural Plast. 2016; 4209831. doi:10.1155/2016/4209831
89. **Umbricht D, Krljes S.** Mismatch negativity in schizophrenia: a meta-analysis. Schizophr Res. 2005; **76**(1): 1–23. doi:10.1016/j.schres.2004.12.002
90. **Umbricht D, Schmid L, Koller R, Vollenweider FX, Hell D, Javitt DC.** Ketamine-induced deficits in auditory and visual context-dependent processing in healthy volunteers: implications for models of cognitive deficits in schizophrenia. Arch Gen Psychiatry. 2000; **57**(12):1139–47.
91. **Berardelli A, Inghilleri M, Rothwell JC, Romeo S, Curra A, Gilio F**, et al. Facilitation of muscle evoked responses after repetitive cortical stimulation in man. Exp Brain Res. 1998; **122**(1):79–84.
92. **Chen R, Classen J, Gerloff C, Celnik P, Wassermann EM, Hallett M**, et al. Depression of motor cortex excitability by low-frequency transcranial magnetic stimulation. Neurology. 1997; **48**(5):1398–403.

93. **Bhandari A, Voineskos D, Daskalakis ZJ, Rajji TK, Blumberger DM.** A review of impaired neuroplasticity in schizophrenia investigated with non-invasive brain stimulation. Front Psychiatry. 2016; 7:45. doi:10.3389/fpsyt.2016.00045
94. **Brody AL, Mandelkern MA, Jarvik ME, Lee GS, Smith EC, Huang JC,** et al. Differences between smokers and nonsmokers in regional gray matter volumes and densities. Biol Psychiatry. 2004; **55**(1):77–84. doi:S0006322303006103 [pii]
95. **Nesvag R, Frigessi A, Jonsson EG, Agartz I.** Effects of alcohol consumption and antipsychotic medication on brain morphology in schizophrenia. Schizophr Res. 2007; **90**(1–3): 52–61. doi:S0920-9964(06)00478-6 [pii] 10.1016/j.schres.2006.11.008
96. **Bangalore SS, Prasad KM, Montrose DM, Goradia DD, Diwadkar VA, Keshavan MS.** Cannabis use and brain structural alterations in first episode schizophrenia—a region of interest, voxel based morphometric study. Schizophr Res. 2008; **99**(1–3):1–6. doi:S0920-9964(07)00530-0 [pii] 10.1016/j.schres.2007.11.029
97. **Konopaske GT, Dorph-Petersen KA, Sweet RA, Pierri JN, Zhang W, Sampson AR, Lewis DA.** Effect of chronic antipsychotic exposure on astrocyte and oligodendrocyte numbers in macaque monkeys. Biol Psychiatry. 2008; **63**(8):759–65.
98. **Konopaske GT, Dorph-Petersen KA, Pierri JN, Wu Q, Sampson AR, Lewis DA.** Effect of chronic exposure to antipsychotic medication on cell numbers in the parietal cortex of macaque monkeys. Neuropsychopharmacology. 2007; **32**(6):1216–23.
99. **Dickerson FB.** Women, aging, and schizophrenia. J Women Aging. 2007; **19**(1–2):49–61.
100. **Antonini G, Mainero C, Romano A, Giubilei F, Ceschin V, Gragnani F,** et al. Cerebral atrophy in myotonic dystrophy: a voxel based morphometric study. J Neurol Neurosurg Psychiatry. 2004; **75**(11):1611–13. doi:75/11/1611 [pii] 10.1136/jnnp.2003.032417
101. **Schizophrenia Working Group of the Psychiatric Genomics Consortium.** Biological insights from 108 schizophrenia-associated genetic loci. Nature. 2014 Jul 24; **511**(7510):421–7.
102. **Stephan AH, Barres BA, Stevens B.** The complement system: an unexpected role in synaptic pruning during development and disease. Annu Rev Neurosci. 2012; **35**:369–89.
103. **Sekar A, Bialas AR, de Rivera H, Davis A, Hammond TR, Kamitaki N,** et al. Schizophrenia risk from complex variation of complement component 4. Nature. 2016 Feb 11; **530**(7589):177–83.
104. **Bitanihirwe BK, Woo TU.** Perineuronal nets and schizophrenia: the importance of neuronal coatings. Neurosci Biobehav Rev. 2014; **45**:85–99.
105. **Cross-Disorder Group of the Psychiatric Genomic Consortium.** Identification of risk loci with shared effects on five major psychiatric disorders: a genome-wide analysis. Lancet. 2013; **381**(9875):1371–9.
106. **Insel TR.** The NIMH research domain criteria (RDoC) project: precision medicine for psychiatry. Am J Psychiatry. 2014; **171**(4):395–7.
107. **Clementz BA**, et al. Identification of distinct psychosis biotypes using brain-based biomarkers. Am J Psychiatry. 2015; **173**(4):373–84.

Chapter 5

Brain changes in psychosis

Understanding their significance as the basis for better prevention

Peter Falkai, Andrea Schmitt, Moritz Rossner, Thomas Schulze, and Nikolaos Koutsouleris

Introduction

Early intervention in mental disorders, including schizophrenia, is based on understanding the underlying mechanisms of the illness. One of the currently pursued pathophysiological hypotheses of schizophrenia is a disturbance of the regenerative capacities of the human brain which leads to disturbed plastic processes [1]. Therefore, strengthening the plasticity of the brain could reduce the likeliness, in schizophrenia, of it developing into a full-blown illness. This chapter puts its focus on structural as well as human post-mortem studies, summarizes the changes described in the literature, and, finally, develops a model from prodromal psychosis to the full picture of schizophrenia with all its underlying structural pathologies.

Neuronal networks involved in psychoses—the hippocampus

A large-scale structural analysis by the Enigma Consortium on patients with schizophrenia and healthy controls demonstrated volume reductions headed by the hippocampal formation, followed by other structures like the thalamus and the basal ganglia [2]. In a recent review [3], five structural imaging studies were identified, comparing prodromal phases of psychosis with healthy controls. Increased volume reduction of the hippocampus could be found in patients with such as cognitive disturbances (COGDIS) and cognitive-perceptive basic symptoms (COPER). Persons showing attenuated psychotic symptoms (APS) or brief limited intermittent psychotic symptoms (BLIPS) demonstrated a larger deficit in verbal memory compared to persons with earlier forms of risk states or genetic risk criterion (i.e. genetic functional risk disorder (GFRD)/COPER). This brings the hippocampus as well as verbal memory into focus as markers for prodromal psychosis [4]. More pronounced structural abnormalities in APS/BLIPS point in the same direction and demonstrate more widespread structural abnormalities— in the medial and lateral temporal lobe structure and the parasylvian prefrontal parietal thalamic and cerebellar regions—associated with basic symptoms (BSs) [5, 6]. When researching the underlying mechanisms, Koutsouleris and co-workers have shown decelerated brain ageing in COPER/GRFD compared to the APs/BLIPS group [7]. They hypothesized that this effect might be due to a maturational delay mechanism or a compensatory neural mechanism at the early stage of the disease. Another working group measured the corpus callosum and the gyrification index for intrahemispheric connectivity [8]. They found impairment in cortico-cortical connectivity, whereas no impaired long-distance connectivity, suggested by a lack of corpus callosum differences, could be supported.

From these studies it can be deduced that in prodromal phases of psychosis, frontotemporal and especially temporal regions are most likely affected, revealing progressive changes from early phases (COPER/GRFD) to later prodromal stages, including psychotic symptoms (APS/BLIPS). This is backed by structural as well as functional data occurring in parallel [4]. For first-episode schizophrenia, this connection between functional and structural impairment of the temporal lobe is supported by a study revealing left hippocampal volume reduction and episodic memory dysfunction determined with a verbal learning and memory test (VLMT) score of 1 to 5 [9]. This leads back to the significance of hippocampal volume reduction as outlined by the large-scale study of the Enigma Consortium [2] mentioned earlier.

Hippocampal volume reduction in schizophrenia

Bilateral volume reduction of the hippocampus in schizophrenia is one of the hallmarks of imaging literature [2], which is partially backed by post-mortem studies [10, 11]. As outlined earlier, such changes cannot only be seen in first- or multi-episode schizophrenia, but in prodromal states of psychosis as well, which consequently brings about the question regarding the nature of these findings.

Bilateral volume reduction of the hippocampus by 4–6 per cent was demonstrated, post-mortem, in schizophrenia patients never treated with antipsychotics [12, 13] and, to the same extent, in patients treated with classical antipsychotics over a long period of time [10]. Using these collected samples of Bogerts and colleagues as a basis for further investigations, we have identified which portion of the neural substrate causes the volume reduction in the hippocampus. By applying unbiased stereological methodology, a reduction of the numbers of macro-neurons could not be demonstrated in schizophrenia [14]. Likewise, as to glia cell populations, no difference in astrocyte numbers could be revealed in schizophrenia, whereas the well-replicated, age-related increase could be replicated [14]. A well-replicated, but yet not undisputed finding in the literature [15] is a significant reduction of interneuron numbers, which we, however, were unable to detect in our sample [16]. On the other hand, a circumscribed reduction of oligodendrocyte numbers was revealed in the CA4/dentate region of the hippocampus [14, 17], which could be shown in the prefrontal cortex by another group as well [18]. Accordingly, electron microscopy analysis demonstrated dystrophy, necrosis, and apoptosis of oligodendrocytes in both regions [19]. Our finding of decreased number of oligodendrocytes was initially described in the posterior portion of the hippocampus, where the subfields are very easily identifiable [14], and were subsequently replicated for the anterior portion of the hippocampus, but only in the left and not the right CA4/dentate region [16]. Staining against parvalbumin and Olig1 and 2, we could find no change of parvalbumin-positive immune reactivity, but did reveal a trend-wise reduction of oligodendrocyte transcription factor (Olig)1, but not Olig2, positive cells [16]. Olig1 antibodies stain precursor forms and mature oligodendrocyte populations, and Olig1 is needed for progenitor development and repair of myelin [20]. This led to the hypothesis that the decreased number of oligodendrocytes is based on a failure of maturation and also indicates a disturbed regenerative process in the CA4/dentate region [1]. Interestingly, this finding is confined to the CA4/dentate region, where neurogenesis can best be observed, and today the CA4 region is regarded as a polymorph layer of the dentate gyrus. Furthermore, this region is the neuroanatomical basis for 'pattern separation' and neurocognitive function shown to be disturbed in schizophrenia [21].

In summary, the major finding of our stereological studies in the hippocampus in schizophrenia is the reduction of oligodendrocytes, probably at their early phase of maturation, in the functionally crucial CA/dentate region. This finding supports the hypothesis of a disturbance of regenerative mechanisms of the human brain in schizophrenia especially affecting neurogenesis and synaptogenesis [1].

Consequently, we attempted to match this finding with clinical symptoms relating to cognitive disturbance. Based on the case notes, we therefore classified patients into either 'possible cognitive deficits' or 'definite cognitive deficits'. Interestingly, the oligodendrocyte reduction was significantly more pronounced in those patients with a definite cognitive deficit [17]. If replicated, this finding could support the idea that disturbed oligodendrocyte integrity might be the basis for cognitive disturbance in schizophrenia. This view is well supported by a number of papers reinforcing the idea that oligodendrocytes provide the key energy supply for axons in the healthy brain [22] and that white matter structures and plasticity have been implicated in cognitive functions and learning [23]. A disturbance in maturation or function of this glial population might well serve as the basis for cognitive dysfunction in neurological (e.g. multiple sclerosis) [24] as well as psychiatric (i.e. schizophrenia) [23] disorders.

Regarding disturbed neurogenesis in schizophrenia, we were able to find reduced volume of the left dentate gyrus and a related reduced number of granule neurons of the left side as well [17]. These findings replicate earlier studies [13, 25] which have described such thinning and which, at the time, had been interpreted as a sign for disturbed neurodevelopment in schizophrenia. More specifically, we would today describe this finding as another sign for disturbed regenerative mechanisms in schizophrenia. Consistent with this finding, decreased cell proliferation in the subgranular zone of the dentate gyrus has been demonstrated and indicates a failure of neurogenesis [26]. However, the oligodendrocyte number reduction—the volume reduction as well as the reduction of the granule neurons in the dentate region—will not account for the 4–6 per cent volume reduction of the hippocampus in general. There is a series of studies available which show, quite nicely, that there is decreased expression of synaptic proteins, especially members of the SNARE (SNAP receptor) complex. The most abundant synaptic protein, SNAP-25, was found to be reduced in expression in the hippocampus, which was interestingly related to a lifelong dysfunction of orientation and judgement in the patients, which could be used as a surrogate marker for cognitive disturbance in schizophrenia [27, 28].

Disturbed brain plasticity—*in vivo* evidence

Based on the post-mortem studies mentioned earlier, one can conclude that schizophrenia is not a classical degenerative disorder but a disturbance of regenerative or plastic processes of the brain [1]. Inspired by animal studies [29], we have performed a three-armed study using physical exercise to improve physical capacity, cognition, and neuronal processes in healthy controls and schizophrenia patients [30]. It could be demonstrated that a three-month regime of indoor cycling, three times a week for 30 minutes each session, could improve verbal memory and increase hippocampal volume by roughly 10 per cent in patients with schizophrenia. Interestingly, these changes could not be found in the control group, where patients played table soccer instead cycling.

In a follow-up study, we then aimed to improve the effect of exercise on brain structure and function in schizophrenia by combining indoor cycling with cognitive remediation [31]. It was possible to demonstrate that the combination of indoor cycling and cognitive remediation improved global functioning (as measured by the global assessment of functioning (GAF) score) by 15 per cent from the baseline to three-month follow-up. It was even more interesting to see that this increase in the GAF score was likewise mirrored in the Social Adjustment Scale (SAS), which showed improvement in the household, social/leisure activities, and general domains. Furthermore, this functional improvement was correlated with an improvement of verbal memory and working memory, which is in line with other studies where improvement in verbal memory has been shown to be a good predictor for positive vocational outcome. When combining table soccer and cognitive rehabilitation, some cognitive improvement in verbal memory could be demonstrated [31]. Researching the effects on the brain of indoor cycling in combination with cognitive remediation revealed an increase of the anterior temporal lobe using voxel-based morphometry. On the contrary, in the table soccer combined with cognitive remediation group, an increase of grey matter was revealed in the anterior cingulate cortex and the premotor area [32].

Meanwhile, two meta-analyses have been published demonstrating a beneficial effect of aerobic exercise on positive but, more especially, negative and global symptoms [33, 34]. Relating the effect of aerobic exercise on cognition, the results are equivocal: one meta-analysis showing a clear-cut effect [34]; the second demonstrating no, or only moderate, effects [33]. Further studies are needed to solve this discrepancy.

When adding neurobiological parameters to the study, there is very little doubt that aerobic exercise seems to improve neuroplasticity of the brain in schizophrenia, accompanied by functional consequences in clinical as well as neurocognitive domains.

Pathophysiological framework for structural changes in psychosis over time

In Fig. 5.1, the identification of the prodrome in psychosis is outlined in the following way. Firstly, an asymptomatic risk state can be identified which is free of symptomatology and characterized by the presence of genetic and non-genetic risk factors. This is followed by an early phase lacking psychotic symptoms (early at-risk mental state: ARMS early) and characterized by a decline of global functioning as well as an increase of affective and basic symptoms (COPER/GRFD). If the prodrome progresses further, there is transformation into a late

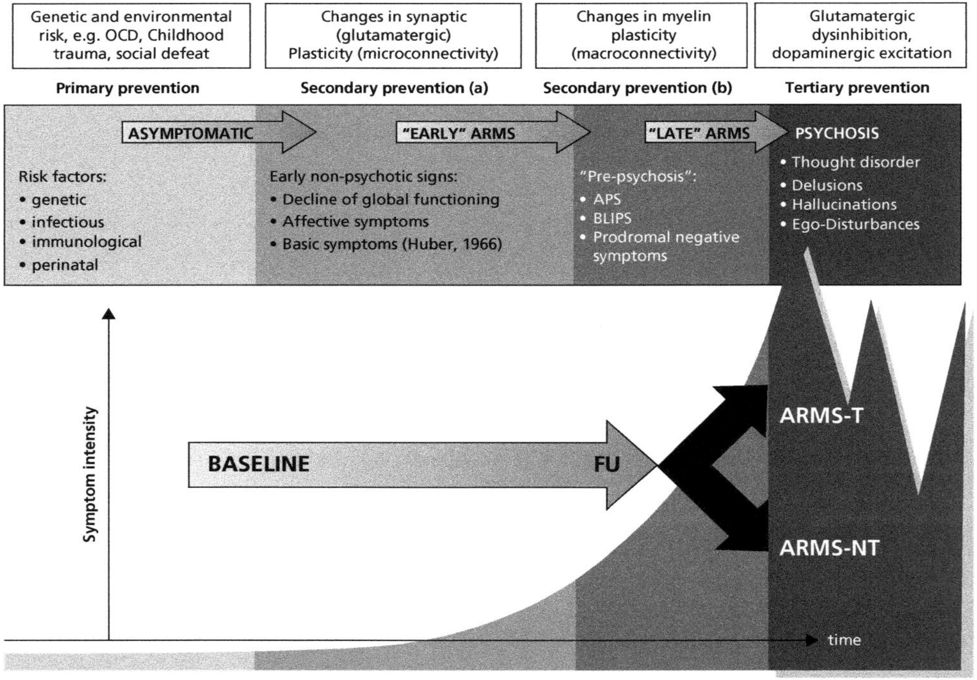

Fig. 5.1 Schematic diagram summarizing, in parallel, the clinical phases of psychotic illness, starting from 'asymptomatic risk state', via 'at-risk mental states', to psychosis and its neurobiological underpinnings.

ARMS-T = persons at an increased risk to develop psychosis (positive family history of psychoses; significant functional decline as determined by the GAF), transiting into psychotic illness within 12 months; ARMS-NT = persons not transiting into psychotic illness within 12 months.

Source data from: Schizophrenia Bulletin, 35, 1, Schultze-Lutter F, Subjective symptoms of schizophrenia in research and the clinic: the basic symptom concept, pp. 5–8, 2009; Häfner H, Maurer K, Löffler W, van der Heiden W, Könnecke R, Hambrecht M. The early course of schizophrenia. Risk and protective factors in schizophrenia—towards a conceptual model of the disease process, pp. 207–228, 2017.

at-risk mental state (ARMS late) phase, revealing APS and BLIPS, as well as prodromal negative symptoms including cognitive dysfunction. Further progression of the prodrome will lead to the full picture of a psychosis demonstrating positive symptoms such as thought disorder, delusions, hallucinations, and ego disturbances, as well as negative symptoms [35, 36].

We hypothesize that the asymptomatic risk state of psychosis is characterized by increased genetic as well as environmental risk load in comparison to the healthy population, but not structural or functional deviations. Persons in anARMS early phase contrarily demonstrate functional as well as structural abnormalities, reaching a degree between the asymptomatic at-risk state and the onset of psychotic symptoms when progressing to the ARMS late phase. The ARMS early phase is defined by a decline of global functioning and an increase of affective and basic symptoms, as outlined earlier. At that stage, several structural abnormalities, especially in the frontotemporal regions, can be detected, compared to healthy controls. It was hypothesized that these changes are due to a failure of synaptic plasticity, specifically targeting the glutamatergic system. The synaptic changes can be primarily due to a failure of synaptic mechanisms or, secondarily, due to a neuronal dysfunction based, for example, on mitochondrial failure causing irregularities of the energy metabolism. Although there is currently no direct evidence for a sequence of events starting from synaptic failure, followed by a disturbance of myelin function, one could deduct the following from existing data. A disturbance of synaptic activity or plasticity will have an impact on neuronal firing or activity. This may subsequently lead to deficits in myelin plasticity, since this process has been shown to be dependent on neuronal activity [23].

Describing the genetic pathways underlying the 108 risk genes for schizophrenia [37], these comprise one for neurodevelopment, one for calcium signalling, one for other ion channels, one for synaptic function and plasticity, and two for glutamatergic and dopaminergic neurotransmission, respectively [38]. It is hypothesized (see Fig. 5.1) that at the ARMS early phase, primarily synaptic changes occur in vulnerable regions (e.g. temporal lobe), targeting glutamatergic mechanisms specifically. These changes are reversible, if the neuronal network is not stressed further on by environmental insults such as cannabis abuse or Bullying. If the illness progresses to the ARMS late phrase, it is hypothesized that, apart from the disturbance of synaptic plasticity, dysfunction of myelin-associated mechanisms also occurs, based on a disruption of oligodendrocyte integrity. These changes are more or less irreversible and lead to cognitive dysfunction, in conjunction with what we call prodromal negative symptoms. If the illness progresses even further, the glutamatergic system becomes more and more inefficient, allowing less control of the dopaminergic system. As the control of the glutamatergic system over the dopaminergic system is lost, step by step, dopamine is released, thus reaching dysfunctional levels and causing positive symptoms. Based on disturbed myelin-associated mechanisms and dysfunction of the glutamatergic system, the full picture of psychosis, with positive as well as negative symptoms, develops (see Fig. 5.1).

Summary of findings and conclusions for improved prevention

Schizophrenia is a complex disorder, where risk genes involved in neuroplasticity are interacting with environmental risk factors like obstetric complications, childhood trauma, social defeat, or cannabis abuse. Schizophrenia and related psychotic illnesses are not degenerative in origin, but are disturbances of regenerative/plastic processes of the brain, involving neurogenetic events in the dentate region, focusing on oligodendrocyte- and synaptogenesis-related processes.

In order to prevent psychosis, persons at risk need to be identified at the early phases of the illness in order to initiate a phase-specific treatment. In ARMS phases, plasticity needs to be boosted (e.g. by aerobic exercise) and risk factors for the brain (e.g. cannabis abuse) need to be reduced or even eliminated. Studies including early ARMS probands have shown that cognitive behavioural therapy (CBT) and antidepressants (ADs) are effective in reducing the likeliness of progression into late ARMS. Once the late ARMS phase is identified, CBT and ADs might well have to be combined with low-dose antipsychotics (APs). However, there are also non-controlled naturalistic studies available which imply that to add an AP will worsen rather than improve the outcome [39]. Well-controlled studies are needed to support this finding.

Once the full picture of the illness has developed, there is no question that APs need to be introduced into treatment, combined with adequate psychotherapy (e.g. CBT, family intervention) and supported employment. However, in order to avoid prodromal psychosis developing into the full clinical state of the illness, it is assumed that plastic processes need to be boosted (e.g. by physical exercise, such as aerobic endurance training, over a period of three months). As we know, these effects are lost in schizophrenia once the intervention is stopped [32]. Either the continuation of aerobic exercise at a reduced strength or the addition of medication (e.g. proglutamateric agents) is therefore needed in order to maintain the plastic effect. On the other hand, stressors—such as cannabis abuse and social defeat (bullying)—must be taken into account,. Consequently, we should improve the plasticity of the brain but also reduce the stress for the brain and the patient.

Altogether, understanding the mechanisms underlying the development of psychosis helps us to develop phase-specific treatment options which, one day, will hopefully allow us to effectively stop the progression of psychosis from the early ARMS phase to full-blown schizophrenia.

References

1. **Falkai P, Rossner MJ, Schulze TG, Hasan A, Brzozka MM, Malchow B**, et al. Kraepelin revisited: schizophrenia from degeneration to failed regeneration. Mol Psychiatry. 2015 Jun; **20**(6):671–6.
2. **van Erp TG, Hibar DP, Rasmussen JM, Glahn DC, Pearlson GD, Andreassen OA**, et al. Subcortical brain volume abnormalities in 2028 individuals with schizophrenia and 2540 healthy controls via the ENIGMA consortium. Mol Psychiatry. 2016 Apr; **21**(4):547–53.
3. **Schultze-Lutter F, Debbane M, Theodoridou A, Wood SJ, Raballo A, Michel C**, et al. Revisiting the basic symptom concept: toward translating risk symptoms for psychosis into neurobiological targets. Front Psychiatry. 2016 Jan 28; 7:9. doi: 10.3389/fpsyt.2016.00009. eCollection;%2016.:9.
4. **Hurlemann R, Jessen F, Wagner M, Frommann I, Ruhrmann S, Brockhaus A**, et al. Interrelated neuropsychological and anatomical evidence of hippocampal pathology in the at-risk mental state. Psychol Med. 2008 Jun; **38**(6):843–51.
5. **Koutsouleris N, Meisenzahl EM, Davatzikos C, Bottlender R, Frodl T, Scheuerecker J**, et al. Use of neuroanatomical pattern classification to identify subjects in at-risk mental states of psychosis and predict disease transition. Arch Gen Psychiatry. 2009 Jul; **66**(7):700–12.
6. **Koutsouleris N, Schmitt GJ, Gaser C, Bottlender R, Scheuerecker J, McGuire P**, et al. Neuroanatomical correlates of different vulnerability states for psychosis and their clinical outcomes. Br J Psychiatry. 2009 Sep; **195**(3):218–26.
7. **Koutsouleris N, Davatzikos C, Borgwardt S, Gaser C, Bottlender R, Frodl T**, et al. Accelerated brain aging in schizophrenia and beyond: a neuroanatomical marker of psychiatric disorders. Schizophr Bull. 2014 Sep; **40**(5):1140–53.
8. **Tepest R, Schwarzbach CJ, Krug B, Klosterkotter J, Ruhrmann S, Vogeley K.** Morphometry of structural disconnectivity indicators in subjects at risk and in age-matched patients with schizophrenia. Eur Arch Psychiatry Clin Neurosci. 2013 Feb; **263**(1):15–24.
9. **Hasan A, Wobrock T, Falkai P, Schneider-Axmann T, Guse B, Backens M**, et al. Hippocampal integrity and neurocognition in first-episode schizophrenia: a multidimensional study. World J Biol Psychiatry. 2014 Apr; **15**(3):188–99.
10. **Bogerts B, Falkai P, Haupts M, Greve B, Ernst S, Tapernon-Franz U**, et al. Post-mortem volume measurements of limbic system and basal ganglia structures in chronic schizophrenics. Initial results from a new brain collection. Schizophr Res. 1990 Oct; 3(5–6):295–301.

11. **van Kesteren C, Gremmels H, de Witte L, Hol A, van Gool A, Falkai P**, et al. Immune involvement in the pathogenesis of schizophrenia: a meta-analysis on post-mortem brain studies. Transl Psychiatry. 2017 Mar 28; 7(3):e1075. doi: 10.1038/tp.2017.4
12. **Bogerts B, Meertz E, Schonfeldt-Bausch R.** Basal ganglia and limbic system pathology in schizophrenia. A morphometric study of brain volume and shrinkage. Arch Gen Psychiatry. 1985 Aug; **42**(8):784–91.
13. **Falkai P, Bogerts B.** Cell loss in the hippocampus of schizophrenics. Eur Arch Psychiatry Neurol Sci. 1986; **236**(3):154–61.
14. **Schmitt A, Steyskal C, Bernstein HG, Schneider-Axmann T, Parlapani E, Schaeffer EL**, et al. Stereologic investigation of the posterior part of the hippocampus in schizophrenia. Acta Neuropathol. 2009 Apr; **117**(4):395–407.
15. **Heckers S, Konradi C.** GABAergic mechanisms of hippocampal hyperactivity in schizophrenia. Schizophr Res. 2015 Sep; **167**(1–3):4–11.
16. **Falkai P, Steiner J, Malchow B, Shariati J, Knaus A, Bernstein HG**, et al. Oligodendrocyte and interneuron density in hippocampal subfields in schizophrenia and association of oligodendrocyte number with cognitive deficits. Front Cell Neurosci. 2016 Mar 30; **10**:78. doi: 10.3389/fncel.2016.00078. eCollection;%2016.:78.
17. **Falkai P, Malchow B, Wetzestein K, Nowastowski V, Bernstein HG, Steiner J**, et al. Decreased oligodendrocyte and neuron number in anterior hippocampal areas and the entire hippocampus in schizophrenia: a stereological postmortem study. Schizophr Bull. 2016 Jul; **42** Suppl 1:S4–12. doi: 10.1093/schbul/sbv157.:S4–S12.
18. **Hof PR, Haroutunian V, Friedrich VL**, Jr., **Byne W, Buitron C, Perl DP**, et al. Loss and altered spatial distribution of oligodendrocytes in the superior frontal gyrus in schizophrenia. Biol Psychiatry 2003 Jun 15;**53**(12):1075–85.
19. **Uranova NA, Vostrikov VM, Vikhreva OV, Zimina IS, Kolomeets NS, Orlovskaya DD.** The role of oligodendrocyte pathology in schizophrenia. Int J Neuropsychopharmacol. 2007 Aug; **10**(4):537–45.
20. **Arnett HA, Fancy SP, Alberta JA, Zhao C, Plant SR, Kaing S**, et al. bHLH transcription factor Olig1 is required to repair demyelinated lesions in the CNS. Science. 2004 Dec 17; **306**(5704):2111–15.
21. **Das T, Ivleva EI, Wagner AD, Stark CE, Tamminga CA.** Loss of pattern separation performance in schizophrenia suggests dentate gyrus dysfunction. Schizophr Res. 2014 Oct; **159**(1):193–7.
22. **Funfschilling U, Supplie LM, Mahad D, Boretius S, Saab AS, Edgar J**, et al. Glycolytic oligodendrocytes maintain myelin and long-term axonal integrity. Nature. 2012 Apr 29; **485**(7399):517–21.
23. **Fields RD.** White matter in learning, cognition and psychiatric disorders. Trends Neurosci. 2008 Jul; **31**(7):361–70.
24. **Kuhlmann T, Miron V, Cui Q, Wegner C, Antel J, Bruck W.** Differentiation block of oligodendroglial progenitor cells as a cause for remyelination failure in chronic multiple sclerosis. Brain. 2008 Jul; **131**(Pt 7):1749–58.
25. **McLardy T, Kilmer WL.** Hippocampal circuitry. Am Psychol. 1970 Jun; **25**(6):563–6.
26. **Reif A, Fritzen S, Finger M, Strobel A, Lauer M, Schmitt A**, et al. Neural stem cell proliferation is decreased in schizophrenia, but not in depression. Mol Psychiatry. 2006 May; **11**(5):514–22.

27. **Barr AM, Young CE, Phillips AG, Honer WG.** Selective effects of typical antipsychotic drugs on SNAP-25 and synaptophysin in the hippocampal trisynaptic pathway. Int J Neuropsychopharmacol. 2006 Aug; **9**(4):457–63.
28. **Young CE, Arima K, Xie J, Hu L, Beach TG, Falkai P,** et al. SNAP-25 deficit and hippocampal connectivity in schizophrenia. Cereb Cortex. 1998 Apr; **8**(3):261–8.
29. **van Praag H., Christie BR, Sejnowski TJ, Gage FH.** Running enhances neurogenesis, learning, and long-term potentiation in mice. Proc Natl Acad Sci U S A. 1999 Nov 9; **96**(23):13427–31.
30. **Pajonk FG, Wobrock T, Gruber O, Scherk H, Berner D, Kaizl I,** et al. Hippocampal plasticity in response to exercise in schizophrenia. Arch Gen Psychiatry. 2010 Feb; **67**(2):133–43.
31. **Malchow B, Keller K, Hasan A, Dorfler S, Schneider-Axmann T, Hillmer-Vogel U,** et al. Effects of endurance training combined with cognitive remediation on everyday functioning, symptoms, and cognition in multiepisode schizophrenia patients. Schizophr Bull. 2015 Jul; **41**(4):847–58.
32. **Malchow B, Keeser D, Keller K, Hasan A, Rauchmann BS, Kimura H,** et al. Effects of endurance training on brain structures in chronic schizophrenia patients and healthy controls. Schizophr Res. 2016 Jun; **173**(3):182–91.
33. **Dauwan M, Begemann MJ, Heringa SM, Sommer IE.** Exercise improves clinical symptoms, quality of life, global functioning, and depression in schizophrenia: a systematic review and meta-analysis. Schizophr Bull. 2016 May; **42**(3):588–99.
34. **Firth J, Stubbs B, Rosenbaum S, Vancampfort D, Malchow B, Schuch F,** et al. Aerobic exercise improves cognitive functioning in people with schizophrenia: a systematic review and meta-analysis. Schizophr Bull. 2017 May 1; **43**(3):546–56.
35. **Häfner H, Maurer K, Löffler W, an der Heiden W, Könnecke R, Hambrecht M.** The early course of schizophreia. Risk and protective factors in schizophrenia—towards a conceptual model of the disease process. In: **Häfner H,** editor. Risk and protective factors in schizophrenia. Heidelberg: Steinkopff; 2017. p. 207–28.
36. **Schultze-Lutter F.** Subjective symptoms of schizophrenia in research and the clinic: the basic symptom concept. Schizophr Bull. 2009 Jan; **35**(1):5–8.
37. **Schizophrenia Working Group of the Psychiatric Genomics Consortium.** Biological insights from 108 schizophrenia-associated genetic loci. Nature. 2014 Jul 24; **511**(7510):421–7.
38. **Schmitt A, Rujescu D, Gawlik M, Hasan A, Hashimoto K, Iceta S,** et al. Consensus paper of the WFSBP Task Force on Biological Markers: criteria for biomarkers and endophenotypes of schizophrenia. Part II: cognition, neuroimaging and genetics. World J Biol Psychiatry. 2016 Sep; **17**(6):406–28.
39. **Fusar-Poli P, Frascarelli M, Valmaggia L, Byrne M, Stahl D, Rocchetti M,** et al. Antidepressant, antipsychotic and psychological interventions in subjects at high clinical risk for psychosis: OASIS 6-year naturalistic study. Psychol Med. 2015 Apr; **45**(6):1327–39.

Chapter 6

Detecting the first signs of emerging psychosis

Frauke Schultze-Lutter

Introduction

Psychotic disorders, particularly schizophrenia, are among the most debilitating illnesses [1, 2]. Although these disorders are commonly diagnosed during the young adult years, and rarely in childhood or early adolescence, schizophrenia is the ninth main cause of disability adjusted life years (DALYs) in 10 to 14-year-old boys, and the second main cause of DALYs in 15 to 19-year-olds of both genders [1]. A prodromal phase of considerable duration commonly precedes the majority of first-episode psychoses, during which decline in psychosocial functioning or delays in the development of psychosocial milestones have already begun to manifest [3]. However, psychoses often remain untreated for extended periods, with prodromal and early psychotic phases together going untreated for an average of over three years, and first-episode psychoses untreated for an average of over one year [4]. These long periods of untreated illness and untreated psychosis are correlated with poor outcome [5]. The delay in treatment is even more pronounced in children and adolescents compared to adults, which may account for the poorer outcome in patients with an age of onset before 18 years compared to those with onset after 18 years [6, 7].

Taken all together, this evidence highlights the need and opportunity for an indicated prevention strategy: an early detection by the first signs of emerging psychosis prior to the first full manifestation. The two dominant approaches to defining clinical high risk of psychosis were developed independent of each other in the 1990s: the ultra-high risk (UHR) approach [8–11] and the basic symptom approach [12–16].

The clinical high-risk criteria for psychosis

Developed in Australia and the United States [8–10], the UHR criteria originated from the observation that, 'although psychotic symptoms are usually viewed as dichotomous events, both patients and nonpatients often report isolated psychotic experiences as well as psychotic-like experiences, the latter being attenuated versions of psychotic experiences ... useful ... especially in studies of individuals believed to be at high risk for future development of clinical psychosis' [17p476]. Such attenuated psychotic symptoms (APS) primarily describe the UHR criteria and account for the majority of inclusions in clinical UHR cohorts [11, 18, 19]. APS encompass the positive features of schizotypal personality disorder (e.g. unusual perceptual experiences, magical thinking/odd beliefs, ideas of reference, suspiciousness/paranoid ideation, odd thinking and speech) which have recently occurred or worsened, and positive symptoms of psychosis (e.g. delusions, hallucinations, formal thought disorders) in which patients still maintain some level of insight. To meet the APS criteria, these phenomena have to deviate significantly from normal and may compromise daily function [8]. Brief intermittent psychotic symptoms (BIPS) that spontaneously resolve, as well as a combination of genetic risk factors (patient has a schizotypal personality disorder and/or a first-degree relative with psychosis) and functional decline, are considered as further UHR criteria. The UHR criteria were explicitly developed to predict the occurrence of first-episode psychosis within 12 months [8, 10] and, thus, focus on symptoms observed in the late prodromal stage (i.e. APS and BIPS) (Fig. 6.1).

In contrast, the basic symptom approach attempts to detect an increased risk of developing psychoses at the earliest possible time, that is, ideally during the initial development of subtle disturbances in information processing [12, 14, 15, 20] (Fig. 6.1). The basic symptom concept was developed in Germany. It originates from retrospective observations of first-episode schizophrenia patients that led researchers to wonder, 'why, hitherto, one has so infrequently made use of the impressive experience that is represented by the first irruption of a thought disorder, a decrease in activity, an aberration in sympathy and other emotions into the healthy personality' [21p296] (translation by the author). Gerd Huber [12, 22] refined the concept and coined the term 'basic' symptom for the assumed close relationship of these symptoms to the neurobiological underpinnings of psychoses [16, 22]. Based on data from a long-term prospective study of patients suspected of developing psychoses [13, 15, 23], two criteria were developed in parallel to the UHR criteria: cognitive-perceptive basic symptoms (COPER) and cognitive disturbances (COGDIS) (see Box 6.1).

An obligate characteristic of the basic symptoms is their subjectivity, that is, the patient's reported experiences of disturbances or aberrations from 'normal' fluctuations in mental state with full and immediate insight [12–15, 24, 25]. Phenomena that might have a somatic cause or result from substance use are not considered basic symptoms. Thus, basic symptoms are qualitatively

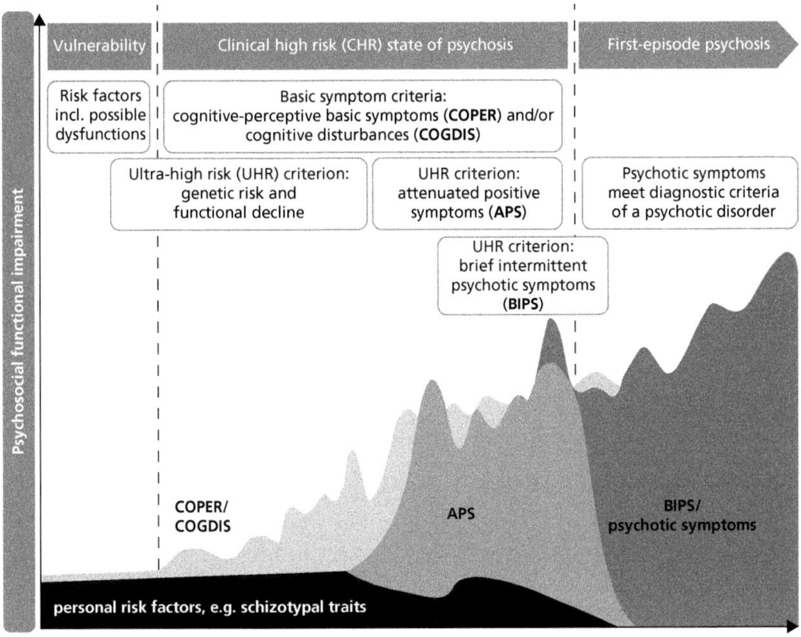

Fig. 6.1 Model of the early course of psychosis.
Source data from: *European Psychiatry*, 18, Schultze-Lutter F, Michel C, Schmidt SJ, et al., EPA guidance on the early detection of clinical high risk states of psychosis, pp. 405–416, 2015; Schizophrenia Bulletin, 32, 4, Fusar-Poli P, Bechdolf A, Taylor MJ, et al., At risk for schizophrenic or affective psychoses? A meta-analysis of DSM/ICD diagnostic outcomes in individuals at high clinical risk, pp. 923–932, 2013.

new in terms of being state markers or significantly increase in frequency while decreasing in their association to situational triggers in terms of being trait-state markers. Consequently, phenomena that have clearly been present throughout life, with the same severity or frequency (trait markers), would not be considered basic symptoms by definition. However, these can be scored as trait characteristics on the Schizophrenia Proneness Instrument in both the adult (SPI-A) [24] and the child/youth version (SPI-CY) [25]. The subtle and self-experienced character of basic symptoms often prevents their detection by others, although coping strategies and emotional reactions related to basic symptoms may be observable. Coping strategies are frequently avoidance strategies, including social withdrawal, while emotional reactions frequently include anxiety and fear related to one's own mental state, as well as feelings of loss of control and helplessness, that might give way to depressiveness [24–26].

Basic symptoms can be clearly distinguished from odd thinking and speech, formal thought disorders, or negative symptoms, which are assessed based

Box 6.1 Basic symptom criteria and definitions of the included symptoms

COGNITIVE-PERCEPTIVE BASIC SYMPTOMS (COPER)

At least any one of the following ten basic symptoms with a SPI-A or SPI-CY score of at least '3' (i.e. at least weekly occurrence) within the last three months *and* first occurrence at least twelve months ago:

Thought interference: Irrelevant, emotionally neutral thoughts with no special meaning, which are not associated with the intended thought, intrude and disturb the young person's train of thought. Yet, the intended thought is not lost.

Thought perseveration: A kind of thought interference in which intruding, emotionally neutral, and irrelevant thoughts or images occur repeatedly.

Thought pressure: A self-reported 'chaos' of thoughts in which successively occurring thoughts are not linked by any common thread and are completely unrelated to each other or to the young person's intended line of thought.

Thought blockages: Sudden interruption in the flow of thoughts, experiences of the mind suddenly going blank, a fading (slipping) of thoughts, or losing the thread of thoughts. The original topic is either lost completely or subsequently recalled.

Disturbance of receptive speech: A disturbance in the understanding of simple everyday words. When reading or listening to others, the young person struggles to comprehend the meaning of words, word sequences, or sentences, even if he or she concentrates on the text or speech and has perceived it accurately.

Decreased ability to discriminate between ideas and perception or fantasy and true memories: A self-recognized difficulty in locating the source of an experience/memory (external vs. internal mental) that results in an inability to immediately distinguish between imagination and perception, or pure fantasy and true memories.

Unstable ideas of reference: Subjective, subclinical experience of self-reference for which no explanation outside one's own mental processes is sought and which is immediately overcome.

Derealization: A change in how one relates emotionally to the environment, which is commonly experienced as an estrangement and detachment from the visual world or, rarely, as an increased emotional affinity for the environment.

Box 6.1 Continued

Visual perception disturbances (excludes blurred vision and hypersensitivity to light): Misperceptions of aspects of the visual field while the young person is fully aware of their true appearance and, therefore, attributes his or her misperception to a problem with eyesight or mental processes.

Acoustic perception disturbances (excludes hypersensitivity to sounds/noises): Misperceptions of acoustic stimuli while the young person is fully aware of the true sound and, therefore, tends to attribute his or her misperception to a problem with hearing or mental processes.

COGNITIVE DISTURBANCES (COGDIS)

At least any two of the following nine basic symptoms with a SPI-A or SPI-CY score of at least '3' (i.e. at least weekly occurrence) within the last three months:

Inability to divide attention: A difficulty in dealing with demands that involve more than one sensory modality at a time and, thus, does not concern demands that would require quick switching of attention.

Captivation of attention by details of the visual field: Domination of the visual field by a random single aspect that captures the young person's whole attention, impedes attention to other aspects, and causes difficulties in turning away from it.

Thought interference (see COPER)

Thought pressure (see COPER)

Thought blockages (see COPER)

Disturbance of receptive speech (see COPER)

Disturbance of expressive speech: A subjective difficulty in verbal fluency and clarity of expression, with words required to express simple ideas being not forthcoming or delayed.

Unstable ideas of reference (see COPER)

Disturbances of abstract thinking: Deficits in the comprehension of any kind of abstract, figurative, or symbolic phrases or content as well as the phenomena of 'concretism' (a limitation of the ability to go beyond the literal meaning of words, sentences, or phrases).

Note: A general requirement of basic symptoms is their novelty (i.e. their report as a disruption in a person's 'normal' self). Self-recognized aberrations in mental processes that have always been present in a trait-like manner can be rated in the SPI-A and SPI-CY (rating of '7'), but are not accounted for as basic symptoms in the strict sense and, consequently, would not contribute to basic symptom criteria.

More in-depth definitions of basic symptoms as well as example questions for the assessment of patients and examples of their statements are provided in the SPI-A and SPI-CY, which can be ordered in various languages from www.fioriti.it.

on communication and other behaviours [24, 25]. Furthermore, since basic symptoms originate within oneself, they are not related to the external world and, consequently, can be distinguished from schizotypy-associated unusual perceptual experiences as well as from hallucinations, which, at least initially, are perceived as real stimuli existing outside and independent of the patient. Finally, since cognitive basic symptoms affect the thought process independent of thought contents, they are clearly distinct from magical thinking, ideas of reference, paranoid ideation, ideas of alien control of thoughts (so called *Ich-Störungen*), or other attenuated or frank delusions that affect thought contents rather than the thought processes themselves [24, 25].

Development of psychosis

According to the basic symptom concept, APS, BIPS, and full-blown psychotic symptoms, which represent the 'end phenomena' of psychotic development, arise after basic symptoms as the result of inadequate coping, including the development of inadequate explanatory models [12]. Thus, unsurprisingly, APS and BIPS are commonly associated with more severe functional impairment [27], more significant neurocognitive impairment [28], and a greater loss of quality of life than basic symptoms [29]. However, the assumption that basic symptoms develop initially, followed by APS, was only partly supported in a retrospective study of 126 first-admission psychosis inpatients, wherein only 86.5% reported prodromal symptoms of some kind (including frequent unspecific basic symptoms) preceding the development of psychotic symptoms [30]. Among the 109 patients with an initial prodromal phase, 50.5% reported basic symptoms of COPER, and 44.9% reported APS. With respect to the sequence of APS and COPER symptoms, among the 58 patients who reported psychosis-risk symptoms, 25 (43.1%) reported a basic symptom of COPER first, 21 (36.2%) reported APS first, and 12 (20.7%) reported co-occurring APS and COPER symptoms [30].

A recent meta-analysis [18] conducted as part of the Guidance Project of the European Psychiatric Association [31] supported the psychosis-predictive utility of both the basic symptom criteria (in particular COGDIS) and the symptomatic UHR criteria (i.e. APS and BIPS). The meta-analysis concluded that there was sufficient evidence to recommend these three criteria as alternative risk criteria for help-seeking patient cohorts. This meta-analysis, which included 42 samples of almost 5,000 patients, revealed pooled conversion rates for COGDIS of 25.3% (95% confidence interval, CI: 22.5–28.1%) at one-year follow-up, which increased to 61.3% (95% CI: 43.9–78.9%) at follow-ups of more than four years (Fig. 6.2) [18]. In comparison, the analysis of the UHR criteria, which was based on a larger number of studies, had pooled conversion rates of 15.0% (95% CI: 12.8–17.1%) at one-year follow-up, that rose to merely 37.0% (95% CI: 33.7–40.2%) at follow-ups of more than four years (Fig. 6.2). Irrespective of their potential for co-occurrence, COGDIS and UHR cohorts did not significantly differ in one- or two-year conversion rates, yet, at three years and beyond, conversion rates in COGDIS cohorts were significantly higher [18] (Fig. 6.2). Thus, this meta-analysis [18], as well as its subsequent replication by Fusar-Poli et al. [19], congruently indicated that basic symptoms, or rather COGDIS, are indeed able to detect an emerging psychotic disorder quite early, even years before its onset, and do so at least as well as the UHR criteria. An earlier meta-analysis [32] also indicated a trend towards higher

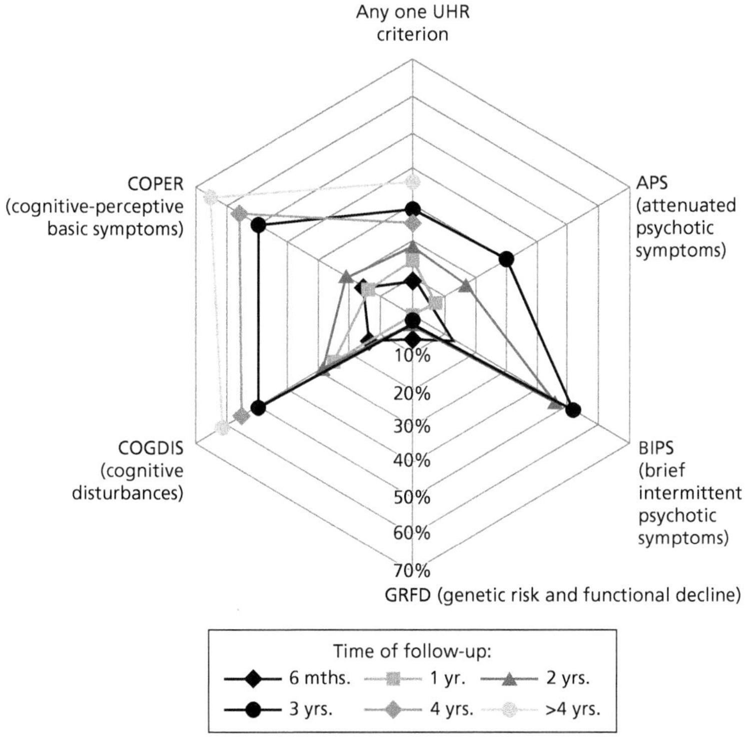

Fig. 6.2 Conversion rates of the different psychosis-risk criteria at different follow-up times: results of a meta-analysis. Note: single criteria might not be exclusive of each other but might co-occur.

UHR, ultra-high risk

conversion rates in studies that included the basic symptom criteria. In addition, a higher rate of conversion to schizophrenia, rather than other psychotic disorders, was observed in basic symptom studies compared to exclusive UHR studies in this meta-analysis [32].

Combining ultra-high risk and basic symptom criteria

Many studies have used either the UHR or basic symptom criteria [18, 19]. However, studies that used both approaches [33–36] consistently reported significantly higher conversion rates in patients who simultaneously met both sets of criteria, mainly APS and COGDIS, than in patients considered at increased risk for psychosis using an exclusive approach. For example, one study examined four-year conversion rates in 246 patients who presented to an early detection service with or without a risk state according to COGDIS and/or symptomatic UHR criteria assessed with the Structured Interview for Psychosis-Risk Syndromes (SIPS) [37]. With a hazard rate of 0.66 at 48 months, the conversion risk of patients meeting a combination of UHR criteria and COGDIS at baseline was approximately 2.5 times higher than that of patients meeting either criterion alone [35]. Here, the hazard rate was 0.28 for patients who met only UHR, and 0.23 for patients who met only COGDIS. By contrast, patients who were not considered at risk only earned an hazard rate of 0.14 at four years. Interestingly, all conversions in the 'only UHR' group occurred within eight months past baseline, while conversions in the 'only COGDIS' group occurred within 6–34 months. The combination group exhibited a steady increase in the conversion rate throughout the four years, which levelled off after 30 months [35]. The authors drew two main conclusions [35], which corroborated other studies [33, 34, 36]. First, the alternative use of symptomatic UHR criteria and COGDIS (i.e. APS/BIPS *or* COGDIS) in the detection of a clinical high-risk state of psychosis considerably increases sensitivity for those who are truly at risk for developing psychosis by detecting those missed using only one approach. Second, the combined use of UHR criteria and COGDIS (i.e. APS/BIPS *and* COGDIS) clearly reduces the risk of false-positive predictions (i.e. it considerably increases specificity). Furthermore, the use of both approaches might provide a stratification of risk in which both the overall risk for conversion and time to conversion might inform the choice of intervention [35].

The value of the combined presence of UHR criteria and basic symptoms was also supported by a recent meta-analysis, although it did not distinguish between the different basic symptom criteria [19].

Psychosis-risk symptoms in the community

From community studies, which were mainly conducted with self-report measures, the median prevalence of psychotic-like experiences was estimated to be 7.2% (0.5–47.2%) [38]. These psychotic-like experiences are frequently assumed to resemble APS [39], and based on these numbers, inclusion of certain psychosis-risk criteria, in particular of attenuated psychosis syndrome, in *DSM-5* was cautioned against since it might pathologize frequent and non-ill experiences in the community. Yet, the mode of assessment seems to play an important role, and self-reporting substantially overestimates the prevalence of APS [38, 40]. Thus, currently very little is known about the prevalence and clinical relevance of psychosis-risk symptoms and criteria in the community when assessed by clinicians in a clinical interview using special instruments. To gain more knowledge, the Bern Epidemiologic At-Risk (BEAR) study [41, 42] and the Bi-National Evaluation of At-Risk Symptoms in Children and Adolescents (BEARS-Kid) study [43, 44] have investigated psychosis-risk symptoms and criteria in community cohorts in a way that is comparable to clinical assessment.

The BEAR study [41, 42] examined different types of psychosis-risk symptoms and criteria, alone and in different combinations, in a large, randomly drawn, representative young-adult community sample (N = 2683; age 16–40; response rate 63.4%) using SIPS and SPI-A, two major instruments for the assessment of psychosis risk in clinical and research settings [45]. Approximately one fifth of participants had experienced psychosis-risk symptoms sometime in their life; three-quarters of those were still experiencing them at the time of the interview [42]. Since risk symptoms were mostly infrequent, they did not meet the frequency requirements of the psychosis-risk criteria. Thus, the prevalence of any psychosis-risk criterion was below the lifetime prevalence rate of psychotic disorders [42], estimated at 3.5% [46] (Fig. 6.3). However, both psychosis-risk symptoms and criteria seem to possess clinical relevance, which is indicated by their significant association with non-psychotic mental disorders and functional deficits [42]. As with the risk of conversion in clinical cohorts, the finding of clinical relevance was highest when UHR and basic symptoms or criteria occurred together. This supports the benefit of their combined use. Furthermore, risk factors described in self-report assessments of psychotic-like experiences [38] were differentially related to UHR and basic symptoms; and only 'first or second-degree relative with a mental disorder' increased the odds for both UHR symptoms and basic symptoms included in COPER and/or COGDIS [42].

In a combined sample of the BEAR and the BEARS-Kid studies [43, 44], which comprised 535 adults aged 18 to 40 years and 154 children and adolescents aged

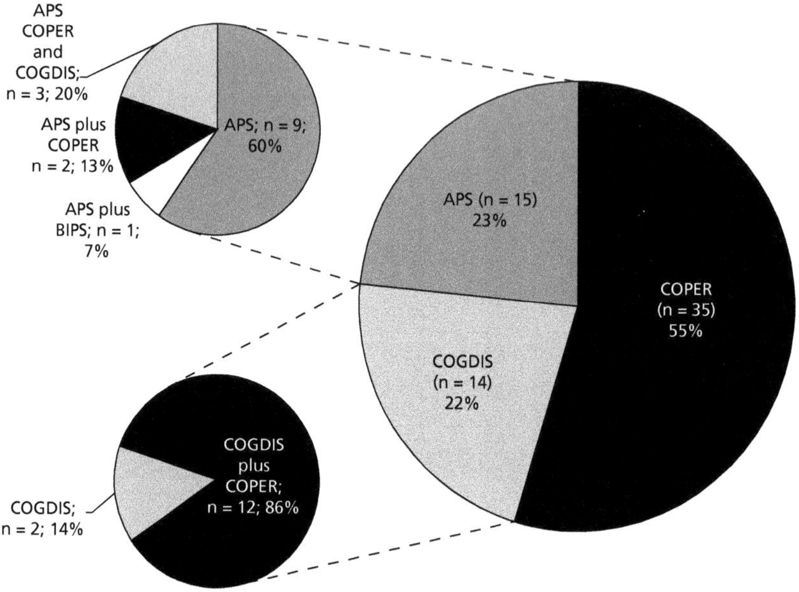

Fig. 6.3 Prevalence and distribution of psychosis-risk criteria in the community (N=2683) according to percentages relating to the 64 participants (2.4%) meeting any one psychosis-risk criterion.

APS, attenuated psychotic symptom criterion of the ultra-high risk criteria; BIPS, brief intermittent psychotic symptom criterion of the ultra-high risk criteria; COPER, cognitive-perceptive basic symptoms; COGDIS, cognitive disturbances.

Reproduced from Early *Interventional Psychiatry*, 10, Schultze-Lutter F, Michel C, Schimmelmann BG., Prevalence of clinical high risk criteria of psychosis in the community: results from the BEAR study. Copyright (2016) with permission from John Wiley and Sons.

8 to 17 years, the influence of age on the prevalence of psychosis-risk symptoms and criteria was studied using the SIPS and SPI-A/SPI-CY. Since high prevalence rates of hallucinatory experiences were reported in children and young adolescents of the community [47], perceptive and non-perceptive symptoms were distinguished [43, 44]. Altogether, 9.9% of the sample reported APS; no participant reported BIPS. Only 1.3% (n = 9) met the APS criterion—seven for perceptive and two for non-perceptive APS [44]. The prevalence of any perceptive APS was 4.9%; that of any non-perceptive APS was 6.1% (6.0% for any unusual thought content, 3.0% for any persecutory idea, 0.3% for any grandiose idea, and 0.7% for any disorganized communication). APS were related to more current axis-I disorders and impaired functioning, indicating some clinical significance. A strong age effect was detected around the age of 16 years: compared to older individuals, 8 to 15-year-olds reported more perceptive APS (i.e. unusual perceptual experiences and attenuated hallucinations). Perceptive

APS were generally unrelated to functional impairment, regardless of age. Conversely, non-perceptive APS were related to low functioning, in particular when their onset was recent. However, this relationship was weak in those below the age of 16 years. Irrespective of their type, APS were also correlated with the presence of a mental disorder; this association was highest in those aged 16 years and above [44]. This age effect and threshold of perceptive APS was recently replicated in a clinical sample of patients from an early detection service [48]. However, in a sample of patients with 22q11 deletion syndrome, age only modulated the prevalence of UHR criteria among those with UHR symptoms, but not the prevalence of APS per se or their clinical significance [49]. The authors regarded this as an indication that patients with 22q11 deletion syndrome might develop early UHR symptoms as a trait factor in terms of a genetically driven schizotypal disposition. However, these symptoms might worsen later on—thereby meeting APS criteria—in those with a higher risk of developing psychosis [49].

With regard to the prevalence of basic symptoms included in COPER and COGDIS, almost twice as many community participants than those reporting APS reported any one of these mainly cognitive, basic symptoms [42]. COPER was reported approximately 2.5 times more often than the APS criterion, while COGDIS was as rare as the APS criterion [42]. Perceptive basic symptoms occurred as infrequently as perceptive APS. Reports of basic symptoms were moderately related to those of APS and, to a lesser extent, more frequent current *DSM-IV* axis-I disorders. Thus, as reported for APS [41, 42], these findings indicated clinical significance of basic symptoms at the community level, with a stronger relation to subthreshold psychotic symptomatology than to non-psychotic disorders [43]. However, the clinical significance of basic symptoms was correlated with age more closely than that of APS, pointing to a differential age threshold at the end of adolescence for perceptive basic symptoms, and another in the early twenties for cognitive basic symptoms [43].

A possible explanation for the varying effects of age on APS and basic symptoms might be offered by the basic symptom concept [12, 14–16]. This concept proposes that basic symptoms are the most direct expression of the underlying neurobiological aberrations, and that APS and psychotic symptoms can be attributed to insufficient coping, including the development of inadequate explanatory models. In light of this, APS would be affected primarily by the development of cognitive abilities, which is largely concluded by late adolescence, while basic symptoms would be affected primarily by brain maturation that continues into young adulthood, particularly in the frontal regions (Fig. 6.4). Thus, APS might be more frequent but less clinically significant at ages before the development of main cognitive abilities is completed, while the same

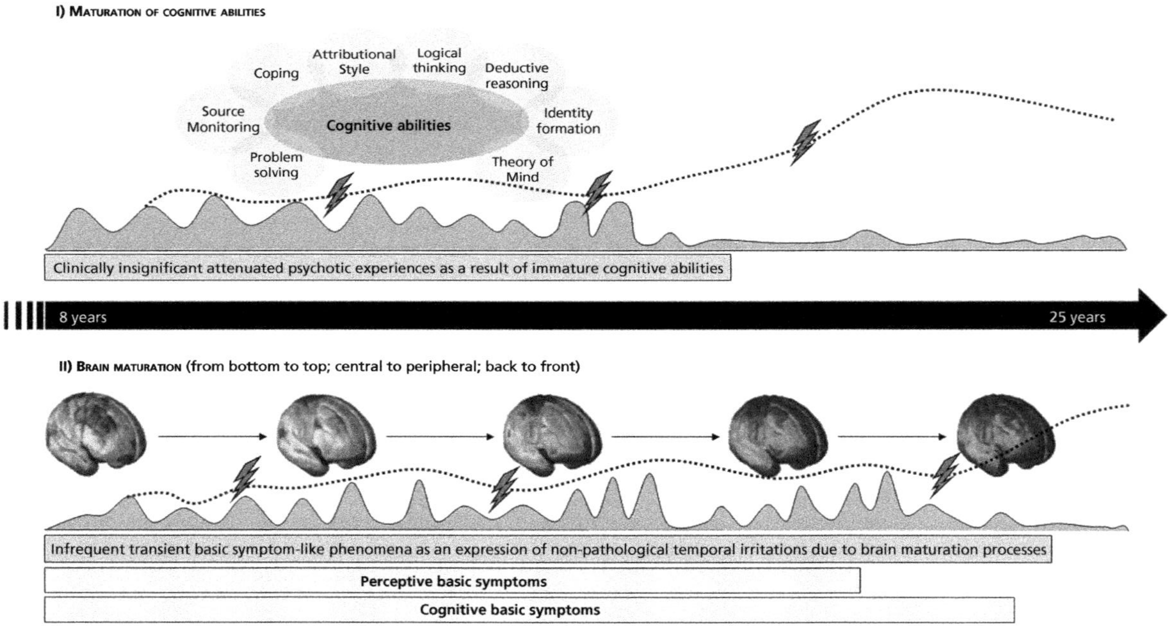

Fig. 6.4 Illustration of the possible relationship between basic symptoms and brain maturation, and attenuated psychotic symptoms (APS) and maturation of cognitive abilities.

This model assumes that (I) unusual perceptual experiences or thought contents identical to APS might occur during childhood and early adolescence as an expression of not yet fully matured cognitive abilities (grey-shaded curve). If their maturation is impaired by risk factors or stressors (flashes) or neurodevelopmental disturbances in information processing, which includes basic symptoms, APS might persist or progress (dotted line), potentially leading to schizotypal traits and/or psychosis. On the other hand, the model assumes that (II) subtle subclinical disturbances in cognitive and perceptive information processing, phenomenologically identical to basic symptoms, might occur during childhood and adolescence as infrequent temporary expressions of minor transient dysfunctions in the wake of brain maturation processes (grey-shaded curve). However, if these disturbances (i.e. basic symptoms) occur more frequently and are persistent (dotted line), they might indicate disturbances in brain maturation which, in line with a neurodevelopmental model of psychosis, predispose the individual to the development of psychosis. A genetic predisposition, childhood adversities, or other risk factors, as well as stressful life events (risk factors/stressors indicated by flashes) and cognitions promoting the development of APS (e.g. poor coping, externalization biases, poor source monitoring) might further fuel the development and persistence of information processing disturbances. Thus, basic symptoms and APS, on concurrence, might reciprocally amplify each other, significantly enhancing the risk of developing psychosis.

Reproduced from *Early Interventional Psychiatry*, 10, Schultze-Lutter F, Ruhrmann S, Michel C, Schmidt SJ, Kindler J, Schimmelmann BG., Basic symptoms in the general population and their association with age. Copyright (2016) with permission from John Wiley and Sons.

might hold true for basic symptoms, in particular cognitive ones, before the conclusion of the maturation of more frontal brain regions [16, 43]. If future studies support this proposed theory, it will provide new important insight into the pathogenesis of psychosis. Furthermore, it will have important therapeutic implications that support the search for effective neuroprotective interventions for basic symptoms, while emphasizing cognitive-behavioural interventions for APS. The combination of both interventions, however, may only be indicated in the group with the highest risk for psychosis (i.e. help-seekers with both APS and COGDIS) [50].

Conclusion

Both UHR and basic symptom criteria (in particular the APS and BIPS criteria) and COGDIS predict psychosis well, especially when used in combination. Thereby, COGDIS (and COPER) might be able to detect emerging psychosis earlier than detected by the symptomatic UHR criteria, which were developed with the explicit aim of detecting first-episode psychosis within the year before its onset.

The idea that psychosis-specific basic symptoms included in COPER and COGDIS occur earlier in the course of psychosis is supported, in part, by retrospective studies on the prodrome of first-episode psychosis, as well as community and clinical risk cohorts, in which those with basic symptoms reported fewer impairments than those with UHR symptoms. Furthermore, since community studies indicated that all psychosis-risk criteria were extremely infrequent, with psychosis-risk symptoms being of some clinical relevance, there is little danger of over-diagnosing the risk of psychosis outside clinical cohorts.

Age, however, needs to be taken into account in the early detection and intervention of psychosis. Furthermore, research into age-related peculiarities of psychosis-risk symptoms will not only support the early detection of psychosis in children and adolescents, but might also support investigations into the origins of psychosis.

References

1. **Gore FM, Bloem PJ, Patton GC, Ferguson J, Joseph V, Coffey C**, et al. Global burden of disease in young people aged 10-24 years: a systematic analysis. Lancet. 2011; 377(9783):2093–102.
2. **Olesen J, Gustavsson A, Svensson M, Wittchen HU, Jönsson B, CDBE2010 study group**. European Brain Council: the economic cost of brain disorders in Europe. Eur J Neurol. 2012; **19**(1):155–62.

3. **Häfner H, Nowotny B, Löffler W, an der Heiden W, Maurer K.** When and how does schizophrenia produce social deficits? Eur Arch Psychiatry Clin Neurosci. 1995; **246**(1):17–28.
4. **Schaffner N, Schimmelmann BG, Niedersteberg A, Schultze-Lutter F.** Versorgungswege von erstmanifesten psychotischen Patienten—eine Übersicht internationaler Studien. Fortschr Neurol Psychiatr. 2012; **80**(2):72–8.
5. **Penttilä M, Jääskeläinen E, Hirvonen N, Isohanni M, Miettunen J.** Duration of untreated psychosis as predictor of long-term outcome in schizophrenia: systematic review and meta-analysis. Br J Psychiatry. 2014; **205**(2):88–94.
6. **Schimmelmann BG, Conus P, Cotton S, McGorry PD, Lambert M.** Pre-treatment, baseline, and outcome differences between early-onset and adult-onset psychosis in an epidemiological cohort of 636 first-episode patients. Schizophr Res. 2007; **95**(1–3):1–8.
7. **Schimmelmann BG, Huber CG, Lambert M, Cotton S, McGorry PD, Conus P.** Impact of duration of untreated psychosis on pre-treatment, baseline, and outcome characteristics in an epidemiological first-episode psychosis cohort. J Psychiatr Res. 2008; **42**(12):982–90.
8. **Yung AR, Phillips LJ, McGorry PD, McFarlane CA, Francey S, Harrigan S**, et al. Prediction of psychosis. A step towards indicated prevention of schizophrenia. Br J Psychiatry, 1998; **172**(Suppl.33):14–20.
9. **Miller TJ, McGlashan TH, Woods SW, Stein K, Driesen N, Corcoran CM**, et al. Symptom assessment in schizophrenic prodromal states. Psychiatr Quart. 1999; **70**(4):273–87.
10. **Phillips LJ, Yung AR, McGorry PD.** Identification of young people at risk of psychosis: validation of personal assessment and crisis evaluation clinic intake criteria. Aust NZ J Psychiatry. 2000; **34**(Suppl):S164–9.
11. **Schultze-Lutter F, Ruhrmann S, Schimmelmann BG, Michel C.** "A rose is a rose is a rose", but at-risk criteria differ. Psychopathology. 2013; **46**:75–87.
12. **Huber G, Gross G.** The concept of basic symptoms in schizophrenic and schizoaffective psychoses. Recenti Prog Med. 1989; **80**(12):646–52.
13. **Schultze-Lutter F, Ruhrmann S, Klosterkötter J.** Can schizophrenia be predicted phenomenologically? In: **Johannessen JO, Martindale B, Cullberg J**, editors. Evolving psychosis. Different stages, different treatments. London, New York: Routledge; 2006: p. 104–23.
14. **Schultze-Lutter F.** Subjective symptoms of schizophrenia in research and the clinic: the basic symptom concept. Schizophr Bull. 2009; **35**:5–8.
15. **Schultze-Lutter F, Ruhrmann S, Fusar-Poli P, Bechdolf A, Schimmelmann BG, Klosterkötter J.** Basic symptoms and the prediction of first-episode psychosis. Curr Pharm Des. 2012; **18**(4):351–7.
16. **Schultze-Lutter F, Debbané M, Theodoridou A, Wood SJ, Raballo A, Michal C**, et al. Revisiting the basic symptom concept: towards translating risk symptoms for psychosis into neurobiological targets. Front Psychiatry. 2016; 7:9.
17. **Chapman LJ, Chapman JP.** Scales for rating psychotic and psychotic-like experiences as continua. Schizophr Bull. 1980; **6**(3):477–89.
18. **Schultze-Lutter F, Michel C, Schmidt SJ, Schimmelmann BG, Maric NP, Salokangas RK**, et al. EPA guidance on the early detection of clinical high risk states of psychosis. Eur Psychiatry. 2015; **30**:405–16.

19. **Fusar-Poli P, Cappucciati M, Borgwardt S, Woods SW, Addington J, Nelson B,** et al. Heterogeneity of psychosis risk within individuals at clinical high risk: a meta-analytical stratification. JAMA Psychiatry. 2016; **73**(2):113–20.
20. **Ruhrmann S, Schultze-Lutter F, Klosterkötter J.** Early detection and intervention in the initial prodromal phase of schizophrenia. Pharmacopsychiatry. 2003; **36**(Suppl 3):162–7.
21. **Mayer-Gross W.** Die Schizophrenie. Die Klinik. In: **Bumke O**, editor. *Handbuch der Geisteskrankheiten*. Berlin: Springer; 1932. p. 293–578.
22. **Huber G.** Reine Defektsyndrome und Basisstadien endogener Psychose. Fortschr Neurol Psychiatr. 1966; **34**:409–26.
23. **Schultze-Lutter F, Klosterkötter J, Picker H, Steinmeyer EM, Ruhrmann S.** Predicting first-episode psychosis by basic symptom criteria. Clin Neuropsychiatry. 2007; **4**(1):11–22.
24. **Schultze-Lutter F, Addington J, Ruhrmann S, Klosterkötter J.** Schizophrenia Proneness Instrument, Adult version (SPI-A). Rome: Giovanni Fioriti Editore; 2007.
25. **Schultze-Lutter F, Marshall M, Koch E.** Schizophrenia Proneness Instrument, Child and Youth version; extended English translation (SPI-CY EET). Rome: Giovanni Fioriti Editore; 2012.
26. **Schultze-Lutter F, Bechdolf A, Wieneke A.** Auf dem Weg in eine schizophrene Psychose? MMW Fortschr Med. 2000; **10**:32–3.
27. **Cotter J, Drake RJ, Bucci S, Firth J, Edge D, Yung AR.** What drives poor functioning in the at-risk mental state? A systematic review. Schizophr Res. 2014; **159**(2–3):267–77.
28. **Frommann I, Pukrop R, Brinkmeyer J, Bechdolf A, Ruhrmann S, Berning J,** et al. Neuropsychological profiles in different at-risk states of psychosis: executive control impairment in the early—and additional memory dysfunction in the late—prodromal state. Schizophr Bull. 2011; **37**(4):861–73.
29. **Ruhrmann S, Paruch J, Bechdolf A,** et al. Reduced subjective quality of life in persons at risk for psychosis. Acta Psychiatr Scand. 2008; **117**:357–68.
30. **Schultze-Lutter F, Rahman J, Ruhrmann S, Michel C, Schimmelmann BG, Maier W,** et al. Duration of unspecific prodromal and clinical high risk states, and help-seeking in prodromal and early psychosis in first-admission psychosis patients. Soc Psychiatry Psychiatr Epidemiol. 2015; **50**:1831–41.
31. **Gaebel W, Möller HJ.** European guidance: a project of the European Psychiatric Association. Eur Psychiatry. 2012; **27**(2):65–7.
32. **Fusar-Poli P, Bechdolf A, Taylor MJ, Bonoldi I, Carpenter WT, Yung AR,** et al. At risk for schizophrenic or affective psychoses? A meta-analysis of DSM/ICD diagnostic outcomes in individuals at high clinical risk. Schizophr Bull. 2013; **39**(4):923–32.
33. **Michel C, Ruhrmann S, Schimmelmann BG, Klosterkötter J, Schultze-Lutter F.** A stratified model for psychosis prediction in clinical practice. Schizophr Bull. 2014; **40**(6):1533–42.
34. **Ruhrmann S, Schultze-Lutter F, Salokangas RKR, Heinimann M, Linszen D, Dingemans P,** et al. Prediction of psychosis in adolescents and young adults—results from a prospective European multicenter study (EPOS). Arch Gen Psychiatry. 2010; **67**(3):241–51.
35. **Schultze-Lutter F, Klosterkötter J, Ruhrmann S.** Improving the clinical prediction of psychosis by combining ultra-high risk criteria and cognitive basic symptoms. Schizophr Res. 2014; **154**(1–3):100–6.

36. **Ziermans TB, Schothorst PF, Sprong M, van Engeland H.** Transition and remission in adolescents at ultra-high risk for psychosis. Schizophr Res. 2011; **126**(1–3):58–64.
37. **McGlashan TH, Walsh B, Woods SW.** *The psychosis-risk syndrome. Handbook for diagnosis and follow-up*. New York: Oxford University Press; 2010.
38. **Linscott RJ, van Os J.** An updated and conservative systematic review and meta-analysis of epidemiological evidence on psychotic experiences in children and adults: on the pathway from proneness to persistence to dimensional expression across mental disorders. Psychol Med. 2013; **43**(6):1133–49.
39. **Schultze-Lutter F, Schimmelmann BG, Ruhrmann S.** The near Babylonian speech confusion in early detection of psychosis. Schizophr Bull. 2011; **37**(4):653–5.
40. **Schultze-Lutter F, Renner F, Paruch J, Julkowski D, Klosterkötter J, Ruhrmann S.** Self-reported psychotic-like experiences are a poor estimate of clinician-rated attenuated and frank delusions and hallucination. Psychopathology. 2014; **47**:194–201.
41. **Schultze-Lutter F, Michel C, Ruhrmann S, Schimmelmann BG.** Prevalence of DSM-5 attenuated psychosis syndrome in adolescents and young adults of the general population: the Bern Epidemiological At-Risk (BEAR) study. Schizophr Bull. 2014; **40**(6):1499–508.
42. **Schultze-Lutter F, Michel C, Ruhrmann S, Schimmelmann BG.** Prevalence and clinical relevance of interview-assessed psychosis risk symptoms in the young adult community. Psychol Med. 2018; **48**:1167–78.
43. **Schultze-Lutter F, Ruhrmann S, Michel C, Schmidt SJ, Kindler J, Schimmelmann BG., Schmidt SJ.** Age effects on basic symptoms in the community: A route to gain new insight into the neurodevelopment of psychosis? Eur Arch Psychiatry Clin. Neurosci. 2018; Epub ahead of print. doi: 10.1007/s00406-018-0949-4.
44. **Schimmelmann BG, Michel C, Martz-Irngartinger A, Linder C, Schultze-Lutter F.** Age matters in the prevalence and clinical significance of ultra-high-risk for psychosis symptoms and criteria in the general population: findings from the BEAR and BEARS-Kid studies. World Psychiatry. 2015; **14**:189–97.
45. **Daneault JG, Stip E, Refer-O-Scope Group.** Genealogy of instruments for prodrome evaluation of psychosis. Front Psychiatry. 2013; **4**:25.
46. **Perälä J, Suvisaari J, Saarni SI, Kuoppasalmi K, Isometsä E, Pirkola S**, et al. Lifetime prevalence of psychotic and bipolar I disorders in a general population. Arch Gen Psychiatry. 2007; **64**(1):19–28.
47. **Schultze-Lutter F, Schmidt SJ.** Not just small adults—the need for developmental considerations in psychopathology. Austin Child Adolesc Psychiatry. 2016; **1**(1):1001.
48. **Schultze-Lutter F, Hubl D, Schimmelmann BG, Michel C.** Age effect on prevalence of ultra-high risk for psychosis symptoms: replication in a clinical sample of an early detection of psychosis service. Eur Child Adolesc Psychiatry. 2017; **26**:1401–5.
49. **Armando M, Schneider M, Pontillo M, Vicari S, Debbané M, Schultze-Lutter F**, et al. No age effect in the prevalence and clinical significance of ultra-high risk symptoms and criteria for psychosis in 22q11 deletion syndrome: confirmation of the genetically driven risk for psychosis? PLoS One. 2017; **12**(4):e0174797.
50. **Schmidt SJ, Schultze-Lutter F, Schimmelmann BG, Maric NP, Salokangas RK, Riecher-Rössler A**, et al. EPA guidance on the early intervention in clinical high-risk states of psychoses. Eur Psychiatry. 2015; **30**:388–404.

Chapter 7

Are ethnic differences in pathways to care for psychosis in England reducing?

Analysis of two population-based studies of first-episode psychosis in South London

Sherifat Oduola, Craig Morgan, and Tom K.J. Craig

Introduction

In the past three decades, there has been a stream of research suggesting that, compared with the majority population, people from minority ethnic groups have a higher incidence of psychosis (e.g. Selten et al. [1], Fearon et al. [2]) and are more likely to come into first contact with mental health services via crisis routes such as emergency departments and police referral [3, 4], and less likely to have general practitioner (GP) involvement in their referral to specialist mental healthcare [5].

Morgan and colleagues, in the Aetiology and Ethnicity in Schizophrenia and Other Psychosis (AESOP) study of 462 FEP patients, reported that, compared with White British, Black Caribbean and Black African patients were less likely to be referred by their GP, but more likely to be referred to mental health services via a criminal justice agency (adj. OR = 1.98, 95% CI 1.04–3.77) [6]. This is consistent with Ghali and colleagues [7] who also reported that Black patients were more likely to be referred to mental health services by a criminal justice agency and less likely to be referred by a GP, compared with White British patients. Interestingly, they found that all ethnic minority patients were more likely to make contact via emergency services [7].

These findings are echoed in other countries. For example, Anderson et al. [8], in a Canadian study of 171 EIS patients, found that Black African patients had an increased odds of contact with the emergency department at first contact (OR = 3.78; 95% CI 1.31–10.92) and Black Caribbean participants had a decreased odds of GP involvement on the pathway to care (OR = 0.17; 95% CI 0.07–0.46) [8].

This predominance of crisis and adversarial pathways and greater use of coercive treatment among minority ethnic groups [9, 10] has been a major source of concern. It was hoped that the introduction of early intervention (EI) services, while not expected to make a difference to inception rates, could make a significant contribution to earlier, less coercive care and so improve outcomes [11, 12].

EI services aim to improve the short- and long-term outcome of psychosis by (a) early detection and reduction in delays to receiving treatment and (b) optimizing medical and psychosocial phase-specific treatments, modified as necessary for use with people at an early stage in the illness [13, 14]. In principle, these services would also reach out to groups of patients known to have difficulty accessing services, perhaps outreaching to emergency rooms in major hospitals or developing contacts with criminal justice agencies, including prison services, to detect and divert patients at an early stage of disorder [15, 16]. Over the last two to three decades, we have seen the establishment of these EI programmes particularly in Western countries, several of which have been carefully evaluated [17–21]. These evaluations show relatively consistent findings of improved clinical and functional outcomes with reduced hospital admissions, relapse rates, and symptom severity, and improved access to care [22]. Perhaps surprisingly, however, very few of these studies have looked at whether these EI programmes have had the desired impact on service access by minority ethnic groups.

In this chapter, we report on our investigations as to whether patients who accessed EI service had reduced likelihood of negative pathways and source of referral during first-episode psychosis, by comparing data from an ongoing incidence study of first-episode psychosis with data from the AESOP study, completed 15 years ago.

Methods

Samples

The two samples were drawn from the same setting in South London, with identical eligibility criteria and measurement of key variables used in the analysis (i.e. source of referral—namely, criminal justice agency, A&E departments, and GP), and identical sociodemographic and pathways to care variables.

Inclusion/exclusion criteria

Inclusion criteria were: (a) resident in the London boroughs of Lambeth or Southwark; (b) aged 18–64 years (inclusive) (16–64 years for AESOP); (c) any psychotic disorder (i.e. ICD F20–29, F30–33); and (d) were making their first contact for psychosis with mental health services. Exclusion criteria were: (a) evidence of psychotic symptom with an organic cause; (b) transient psychotic symptoms resulting from acute intoxication; and (c) evidence of previous contact with services for psychotic symptoms.

At the time of the CRIS-FEP (Clinical Records Interactive Search–First-Episode Psychosis) study, the age eligibility criteria for early intervention services (EIS) in South London and Maudsley (SLaM) were 18–35 years. Therefore, data from the CRIS-FEP and the AESOP studies for this report were restricted to patients aged 18–35 years. In addition, the following ethnic groups—White British, Black African, Black Caribbean, and White Other—have been reported to experience more problematic pathways to care. To that end, for the purpose of analysis, we restricted data from both CRIS-FEP and AESOP studies to these groups. This enabled us to make direct comparisons between the two study samples.

Study design, setting, and participants

The methods used in the AESOP study have been widely published elsewhere [2, 3]. Briefly, it was a three-centre study in South London, Nottingham, and Bristol, in which individuals with any psychotic disorder (i.e. ICD F20–29, F30–33) were identified through liaison between the study team and the mental health services in the study catchment areas. For this chapter, we include only cases from the AESOP London site.

The CRIS-FEP study is a case-register study of first-episode psychosis. All patients presenting to SLaM NHS Trust adult mental health services in Lambeth and Southwark, for the first time, with a psychotic disorder (including F20–29 and F30–33 in the *ICD 10*), between May 2010 and April 2012, were identified. Data were drawn from the SLaM NHS Trust CRIS system [23], with a three-stage manual screening of clinical records by a team of researchers. Firstly, symptom terms (including psychos*, psychot*, delusion*, voices, hallucinat*, paranoia), service location (i.e. Lambeth and Southwark), diagnosis, and age range were applied to the CRIS, using structured query language (SQL) commands [24], on a weekly basis. This returned a set of patient records, which were individually screened by a team of researchers using the Psychosis Screening Schedule [25]. Researchers swapped cases and rescreened for inter-rater reliability; an 87.4% agreement, along with a kappa score of 0.78 ($p < 0.01$), was achieved. Secondly, two primary researchers reviewed all the included cases from the first-stage screen to ensure cases met all inclusion criteria. Thirdly, discrepant or ambiguous cases were resolved by consensus with the principal investigator (CM).

Ethnicity was self-ascribed and recorded in clinical records. Where this information was missing, ethnicity was ascribed independently by researchers using all available information from the clinical records, including country of birth, nationality, language spoken at home, and parents' country of birth (as recommended by the Office of National Statistics [26]). High inter-rater reliability was achieved between three researchers; each independently extracted ethnicity information on 89 cases (kappa score of 0.87, $p < 0.001$).

Data were collected on sociodemographic variables using the Medical Research Council Sociodemographic Schedule MRC-SDS [27]. Data relating to source of referral, pathways to care, and the duration of untreated psychosis were collected using a modified form of the Personal and Psychiatric History Schedule (PPHS) [28] for the purpose of data collection from case notes.

Statistical analysis

Data were analysed using Stata version 12 [29]. First, we used logistic regression to assess unadjusted associations between sociodemographic and pathways to care variables and each primary outcome (i.e. GP, police or criminal justice agency, and emergency referrals). Second, we adjusted all analyses for a priori potential confounders (age, gender, and employment status) to control for demographic and socioeconomic status. Third, we then added other variables that were crudely associated with the outcome variables from the univariable analyses; we included variables if the p-value was ≤0.05.

For the AESOP study, ethical approval was provided in all sites. The CRIS system was approved as an anonymized dataset for secondary analysis by the Oxfordshire Research Ethics Committee (reference 08/H0606/71). Local approval for this study was obtained from the CRIS Oversight Committee at the BRC (Biomedical Research Centre) SLaM NHS Foundation Trust (reference 09-041).

Results

A total of 278 first-episode psychosis patients at the London site were part of the AESOP study, of whom 193 were aged 18–35 years and were thus included for the current analysis. From the CRIS-FEP study, a total of 558 first-episode patients were identified, of whom 265 were 18–35 years and thus would have been eligible for EIS services. Of these, 184 received care from an EIS.

Of the 81 patients who were eligible for EIS care but did not access it, 25 (29.7%) were seen in other specialist services (i.e. perinatal, mother and baby unit, HIV service, and forensic services), but the remainder were managed throughout in generic community mental health/outpatient services, despite the well-established EIS pathway for first-episode care.

Table 7.1 shows the demographic and pathways to care variables for AESOP and CRIS-FEP, with the latter separated by whether or not the patient received care from a specialist EIS team. Compared with AESOP, Black Caribbean patients comprise a smaller, and Black African patients a larger, proportion of the CRIS-FEP total sample, and there was a somewhat greater proportion of people with higher or university-level education. The proportion of patients accessing services via police and criminal justice agencies was also substantially lower than observed in AESOP. Furthermore, a higher proportion of patients in the CRIS-FEP sample accessed services through the accident and emergency route compared with AESOP. More differences emerged when the CRIS-FEP sample was broken down by receipt of EIS. It is apparent that the patients who were seen by EIS were somewhat younger, more likely to be men, educated to university level, lived with family, and to have family involvement in their pathway to care than either patients in AESOP or those who were eligible for EIS but did not receive it.

In the AESOP sample, Black African (OR = 0.29; 95% CI = 0.12–0.70, $p < 0.01$) and Black Caribbean (OR = 0.45; 95% CI = 0.21–0.95, $p = 0.05$) patients were less likely to be referred to mental health services by their GP. Interestingly, associations between GP referral and ethnicity in the CRIS- FEP sample differed by whether or not the patient had contact with EIS. In the non-EIS group, and similar to AESOP, Black Caribbean patients were less likely to access care via their GP (OR = 0.17; 95% CI = 0.03–0.93, $p = 0.04$), but the evidence was weak for Black African patients (OR = 0.32; 95% CI = 0.09–1.16, $p = 0.08$). By contrast, the subgroup that was seen in EIS showed no association between ethnicity and GP referral. Those with longer duration of untreated psychosis were over two times more likely to be referred by a GP (OR = 2.60; 95% CI = 1.34–5.05 $p < 0.01$).

When we examined the associations between sociodemographic and pathways to care variables and A&E referral, there was strong evidence that those who had family involvement in their pathways to care were more likely to seek help via A&E services; this was notable in both the AESOP (OR = 3.64; 95% CI = 1.91–6.91, $p < 0.01$) and CRIS-FEP (non-EIS, OR = 4.48; 95% CI = 1.63–12.32, $p < 0.04$ and EIS, OR = 5.23; 95% CI = 2.72–9.91, $p < 0.01$) samples. There was no evidence of associations between other variables and emergency referral in the AESOP sample. In the non-EIS group, Black Caribbean patients were four times more likely to come into contact with mental health services via an A&E route (OR = 4.04; 95% CI = 1.05–15.47, $p = 0.04$). In the EIS group,

Table 7.1 Demographic and pathways to care characteristics of AESOP and CRIS-FEP samples

	AESOP	CRIS-FEP	
	AESOP N=193 (%)	**Non-EIS N=81 (%)**	**EIS N=184 (%)**
DEMOGRAPIC VARIABLES			
Mean age (sd) years	26.7 (4.9)	27.5 (5.0)	25.5 (5.1)
Gender			
Men	110 (57.0)	38 (46.9)	116 (63.0)
Women	83 (43.0)	43 (53.1)	68 (37.0)
Ethnicity			
White British	60 (31.1)	23 (28.4)	55 (29.9)
Black African	50 (25.9)	25 (30.9)	70 (38.1)
Black Caribbean	65 (33.7)	17 (21.0)	35 (19.0)
White Other	18 (9.3)	16 (19.7)	24 (13.0)
Education[1]			
School, no GCSE	51 (27.6)	23 (35.4)	27 (18.9)
School, GCSE	46 (24.8)	11 (16.9)	28 (19.6)
Further	57 (30.8)	15 (23.1)	45 (31.4)
Higher/University	31 (16.8)	16 (24.6)	43 (30.1)
Employment[2]			
Unemployed	112 (59.0)	56 (73.7)	101 (58.4)
Student/Other	24 (12.6)	7 (9.2)	39 (22.5)
Employed	54 (28.4)	13 (17.1)	33 (19.1)
Relationship status[3]			
Single	124 (70.1)	55 (71.4)	123 (69.1)
Married/In steady relationship	42 (23.7)	17 (22.1)	41 (23.0)
Divorced/Widowed	11 (6.2)	5 (6.5)	14 (7.9)
Living arrangements[4]			
Alone	86 (45.0)	25 (31.6)	34 (18.8)
Family/ Relatives	90 (47.1)	42 (53.2)	126 (69.6)
Other	15 (7.9)	12 (15.2)	21 (11.6)

Table 7.1 Continued

	AESOP	CRIS-FEP	
	AESOP N=193 (%)	**Non-EIS N=81 (%)**	**EIS N=184 (%)**
PATHWAYS TO CARE VARIABLES			
DUP[5]			
Short (≤ 1 year)	157 (81.4)	61 (75.3)	129 (70.1)
Long (> 1 year)	36 (18.6)	20 (24.7)	55 (29.9)
Family involvement in help-seeking[6]			
Yes	65 (35.5)	25 (30.9)	86 (46.7)
No	118 (64.5)	56 (69.1)	93 (53.3)
GP referral[7]			
No	129 (67.2)	59 (72.8)	125 (67.9)
Yes	63 (32.8)	22 (27.2)	59 (32.1)
A&E referral[8]			
No	127 (66.1)	46 (56.8)	108 (58.7)
Yes	65 (33.9)	35 (43.2)	76 (41.3)
Police/CJA referral[9]			
No	141 (73.4)	71 (87.7)	156 (84.8)
Yes	51 (26.6)	10 (12.3)	28 (15.2)

Missing data

1. AESOP, 8; CRIS-FEP, 57 (EIS = 41; non-EIS = 16)
2. AESOP, 3; CRIS-FEP, 16 (EIS = 11; non-EIS = 5)
3. AESOP, 16; CRIS-FEP, 10 (EIS = 6; non-EIS = 4)
4. AESOP, 2; CRIS-FEP, 5 (EIS = 3; non-EIS = 2)
5. AESOP, none; CRIS-FEP, none
6. AESOP, 10; CRIS-FEP, none

7–9. AESOP, 1; CRIS-FEP, none

compared with those educated to university level, patients without school qualifications were less likely to access services via the A&E route (OR = 0.29; 95% CI = 0.10–0.88, p = 0.03).

For the relationship between sociodemographic and pathways to care variables and criminal justice agency referral, two variables were relevant in the AESOP sample: namely, age (OR = 1.11; 95% CI = 1.03–1.19, p < 0.01) and ethnicity (Black African, OR = 4.55; 95% CI = 1.62–12.71 and Black Caribbean, OR = 5.52; 95% CI = 2.06–14.72, p < 0.01). As would be expected, those who had family involvement in their help-seeking were less likely to be referred by the criminal justice agency (OR = 0.20; 95% CI = 0.08–0.49, $p < 0.01$). This was mirrored in the EIS group (OR = 0.15; 95% CI = 0.04–0.45, $p < 0.01$).

When we repeated the analyses and adjusted for possible confounders, including demographic, socioeconomic, duration of untreated psychosis, and family involvement in help-seeking variables, the findings on GP referral for Black Caribbean and Black African patients in the AESOP sample held (i.e. adj. OR = 0.37; 95% CI = 0.15–0.92 and adj. OR = 0.24; 95% CI = 0.08–0.70, respectively). However, the results on GP referral for Black Caribbean were less robust in the non-EIS group (adj. OR = 0.18; 95% CI = 0.01–2.42).

The robust associations between criminal justice agency referral and Black Caribbean and Black African patients remained in the adjusted analysis in the AESOP sample, and showed that both ethnic groups were still eight and four times more likely than White British patients to be referred by the criminal justice agency (adj. OR = 8.16; 95% CI = 2.45–26.20, $p < 0.01$ and adj. OR = 4.30; 95% CI = 1.28–14.45, $p = 0.03$, respectively). These associations were independent of the a priori confounders as well as duration of untreated psychosis and family involvement variables.

Further, the striking differences observed for A&E referral in the non-EIS sample also held for Black Caribbean and Black African patients. For example, after adjusting for demographic, socioeconomic status, duration of untreated psychosis (DUP), and family involvement variables, Black Caribbean and Black African patients were substantially more likely than White British to be referred via A&E (adj. OR = 48.89; 95% CI = 3.49–684.71; $p < 0.01$, and adj. OR = 7.34; 95% CI = 1.15–46.74; $p = 0.03$, respectively). The findings for the Black Caribbean group, in particular, need to be treated cautiously, given the very wide confidence intervals. The findings for White Other patients were less robust (Table 7.2).

Discussion

Main findings

This study, using two independent population-based samples, suggests that changes have occurred in the pathways to care for people with first-episode psychosis. Compared with 15 years ago, a greater proportion of users of EIS have family involvement in their pathway to care. Ethnic differences were not evident for problematic pathways to care involving the police and criminal justice agency, regardless of EIS status. Further, both Black Caribbean and Black African patients are now comparable to White British patients in the involvement of their GP on the pathway to care in both EIS and non-EIS groups. However, many patients who met the criteria for EIS did not access them. The

Table 7.2 Adjusted odds ratios of associations between ethnicity and source of referral, by use of EIS

	AESOP Adjusted odds ratios (95% CI)			**CRIS-FEP: non-EIS group Adjusted odds ratios (95% CI)**			**CRIS-FEP: EIS group Adjusted odds ratios (95% CI)**		
	GP referral	**A&E referral**	**CJA referral**	**GP referral**	**A&E referral**	**CJA referral**	**GP referral**	**A& E referral**	**CJA referral**
Ethnicity									
White British	Reference	Reference	Reference	Reference	Reference	Reference	Reference	Reference	Reference
Black African	0.24 (0.08–0.70)**	1.14 (0.44–2.94)	4.30 (1.28–14.45)**	0.37 (0.71–2.00)	7.34 (1.15–46.74)*	0.26 (0.01–4.09)	0.57 (0.20–1.62)	1.98 (0.71–5.48)	1.35 (0.35–5.20)
Black Caribbean	0.37 (0.15–0.92)*	0.56 (0.23–1.40)	8.16 (2.54–26.20)**	0.18 (0.01–2.42)	48.89 (3.49–684.71)**	No cases	1.20 (0.37–3.87)	0.75 (0.22–2.55)	1.06 (0.16–7.01)
White Other	1.13 (0.32–3.97)	0.97 (0.24–3.82)	1.24 (0.23–6.55)	0.97 (0.14–6.62)	7.03 (0.78–62.76)†	0.06 (0.00–3.82)	1.14 (0.32–4.04)	1.74 (0.48–6.32)	1.14 (0.14–8.73)

Adjusted for: age, gender, employment status, family involvement, education level and DUP

† P=0.1; * p≤0.05 ** p≤0.01

CJA, criminal justice agency; A&E, accident and emergency; GP, general practitioner; CI, confidence intervals.

results in our non-EIS group showed that all the minority ethnic groups (albeit only slightly for the White Other ethnic group) were more likely than White British patients to access care through A&E services. The evidence suggests that these differences may not be driven by ethnicity alone but perhaps influenced by social factors (such as the involvement of significant others in help-seeking). The findings also indicate that family play a crucial role in help-seeking, particularly during acute onset of psychosis when help may be required urgently.

Methodological considerations

Since the completion of the AESOP study, the CRIS-FEP study is one of the largest studies of first-episode psychosis. The key strengths in this study are its large sample sizes and the comparison of two datasets collected in the same study area at different time points. These allowed the investigation of ethnic differences in pathways to care at two time points in South London.

The cross-sectional nature of our data means that the differences in associations between ethnicity and pathways to care in the two samples may not be explained by the introduction of EIS alone; it could be due to other factors. While we adjusted for demographic, socioeconomic, and pathways to care variables, our study may still be confounded by unmeasured variables. Further, the loss of power in the adjusted analyses means that the observed positive associations may be due to chance. For example, the small sample size in the non-EIS group and wide confidence interval around the elevated odds ratios for minority ethnic status and A&E referral are interpreted tentatively.

The difference in the proportion of patients experiencing a long (≥ 1 year) DUP (28.3% in the CRIS-FEP study compared with 18% of the AESOP sample) potentially highlights some methodological considerations in the case-identification process used in the AESOP study. Given the shorter duration of psychosis experienced by the AESOP sample, it is possible that cases with a long DUP may have been missed, especially if patients were predominantly identified in hospital or community crisis services.

Despite the comprehensive case finding in the CRIS-FEP study, it is important to note that data were recorded by clinicians for clinical purposes, and not collected for research; therefore, the accuracy of information depends on the quality of clinicians' notes. In addition, if information is not recorded, it is not known if it is simply not available.

Relationship to previous studies

Our data on source of referral and pathways to care suggest that the way people make contact with and seek help from mental health services may have changed compared with some previous studies. Many previous studies have reported that Black African and Black Caribbean patients were more likely to come in contact with services via the criminal justice system [7, 30]. This study is one of the few to find no ethnic differences in criminal justice agency referral at first contact with services [10]. In both EIS and non-EIS samples, the proportions of Black Caribbean (14.3% and 11.7% respectively) and Black African (18.6% and 12.0% respectively) patients referred via the criminal justice system were similar to those of White British patients (14.5% and 17.4% respectively). These proportions are much lower than those we found in the AESOP sample here, and even lower than those reported in previous studies. Evidence of lower levels of GP involvement among the Black Caribbean group was partly consistent with previous research [5, 8]. However, our findings of increased risk for criminal justice agency referral among Black African and Black Caribbean patients in the AESOP sample are consistent with other studies [30, 31] and with reduced likelihood of GP referral among the same ethnic groups [7]. The findings on A&E referral, that showed Black African and Black Caribbean patients were more likely to be referred to mental health services via this route, are consistent with previous research [4, 32]. We did not find associations between ethnic minority status and A&E referral in the AESOP sample.

Interestingly, socioeconomic position and involvement of family in pathways to care appear to play a key role in explaining the increased likelihood of minority ethnic group and A&E referral. Several authors have argued that careful consideration must be given to socioeconomic status in studies investigating the relationship between ethnicity and mental health. Considering our non-EIS sample, unemployment and poor education were higher compared with EIS and AESOP samples. It is possible that the previously suggested explanation of poor understanding of help-seeking among minority ethnic groups may also explain this difference [33–35]. However, this may be difficult to disentangle since psychosis is linked to behavioural problems and affects relationships and executive functioning, which may possibly precede unemployment or lack of education qualifications, and indeed vice versa.

It is noteworthy that an AESOP leakage study was conducted to identify any cases missed through the routine procedures; this accounted for 14.3% of the sample [2, 3]. Case identification in the CRIS-FEP study points to a more comprehensive search for psychosis cases, since by screening the multidisciplinary healthcare professional documented clinical records, we were able to identify more persons with clear psychotic features within the study catchment area.

A key source of concern is that 81 of the CRIS-FEP patients who were eligible for EIS did not receive it. This violates the National Institute for Clinical Excellence recommendation that adults with a first episode of psychosis (FEP) should start treatment in EIS within two weeks of referral [36]. Reiterating the difference in the proportions of patients with DUP of more than a year, particularly among the non-EIS group, may shed some light on possible explanations for this group not reaching EIS. A long DUP in our non-EIS group was evident for 25%, compared with 18% in the AESOP sample. In addition, data on the type of service use for the non-EIS group showed that the majority of patients were receiving care from specialist mental health services (i.e. perinatal, mother and baby unit). This may suggest that these patients may have experienced other disorders prior to the manifestation of psychosis and, therefore, these services continue to treat them for the initially recognized disorder as well as for psychosis. This is a plausible explanation, since there were mostly women in our non-EIS group. However, delays in reaching EIS have been previously reported. Birchwood and colleagues, in a cross-sectional study of DUP and care pathways, sought to investigate DUP and its link with delays in accessing specialist EIS [37]. In a sample of 343 patients recruited from an EIS, they found an overall mean DUP of 260 days. However, a third of the sample had a DUP greater than six months; these were patients whose first contact with mental health services was generic care (e.g. community mental health team). The researchers found that delay in reaching EIS was strongly correlated with longer DUP.

Conclusions

Our findings suggest that the disparities in pathways to care between White British and minority ethnic group patients seem to be narrowing. However, there appears to be ethnic differences in contact via hospital A&E rooms. Socioeconomic factors and family involvement in the pathways to care may be important in explaining ethnic differences in those accessing A&E services.

References

1. **Selten JP, Veen N, Feller W, Blom JD, Schols D, Camoeniě W**, et al. Incidence of psychotic disorders in immigrant groups to the Netherlands. Br J Psychiatry. 2001 Apr; **178**:367–72.
2. **Fearon P, Kirkbride JB, Morgan C, Dazzan P, Morgan K, Lloyd T**, et al. Incidence of schizophrenia and other psychoses in ethnic minority groups: results from the MRC AESOP Study. Psychol Med. 2006; **36**(11):1541–50.
3. **Morgan C, Mallett R, Hutchinson G, Bagalkote H, Morgan K, Fearon P**, et al. Pathways to care and ethnicity. 2: Source of referral and help-seeking. Report from the AESOP study. Br J Psychiatry. 2005; **186**:290–6.
4. **Anderson K, Fuhrer R, Malla A.** The pathways to mental health care of first-episode psychosis patients: a systematic review. Psychol Med. 2010; **40**(10):1585–97.

5. **Bhui K,Bhugra D.** Mental illness in Black and Asian ethnic minorities: pathways to care and outcomes. Adv Psychiatr Treat. 2002; **8**(1):26–33.
6. **Morgan C, Mallett R, Hutchinson G, Bagalkote H, Morgan K, Fearon P**, et al. Pathways to care and ethnicity. 1: Sample characteristics and compulsory admission. Report from the AESOP study. Br J Psychiatry. 2005; **186**:281–9.
7. **Ghali S, Fisher HL, Joyce J, Major B, Hobbs L, Soni S**, et al. Ethnic variations in pathways into early intervention services for psychosis. Br J Psychiatry. 2013; **202**(4);277–83.
8. **Anderson KK, Archie S, Boursiquot PE, Buffett J, Canso D, Ferrari M**, et al. Pathways to first-episode care for psychosis in African-, Caribbean-, and European-origin groups in Ontario. Can J Psychiatry. 2015; **60**(5):223–31.
9. **Ouellet-Plamondon C, Rousseau C, Nicole L, Abdel-Baki A.** Engaging immigrants in early psychosis treatment: a clinical challenge. Psychiatr Serv. 2015; **66**(7):757–9.
10. **Burnett R, Mallett R, Bhugra D, Hutchinson G, Der G, Leff J**, et al. The first contact of patients with schizophrenia with psychiatric services: social factors and pathways to care in a multi-ethnic population. Psychol Med. 1999; **29**(2):475–83.
11. **Mann F, Fisher HL, Johnson S.** A systematic review of ethnic variations in hospital admission and compulsory detention in first-episode psychosis. J Ment Health. 2014; **23**(4):205–11.
12. **Marshall M, Lewis S, Lockwood A, Drake R, Jones P, Croudace T.** Association between duration of untreated psychosis and outcome in cohorts of first-episode patients: a systematic review. Arch Gen Psychiatry. 2005;**62**(9):975.
13. **Marshall M, Rathbone J.** Early intervention for psychosis. Schizophr Bull. 2011; **37**(6):1111–14.
14. **Joseph R, Birchwood M.** The national policy reforms for mental health services and the story of early intervention services in the United Kingdom. J Psychiatry Neurosci. 2005; **30**(5):362.
15. **Jarrett M, Craig T, Parrott J, Forrester A, Winton-Brown T, Maguire H**, et al. Identifying men at ultra high risk of psychosis in a prison population. Schizophr Res. 2012;**136**(1):1–6.
16. **Fusar-Poli P, Byrne M, Badger S, Valmaggia LR, McGuire PK.** Outreach and support in South London (OASIS), 2001–2011: ten years of early diagnosis and treatment for young individuals at high clinical risk for psychosis. Eur Psychiatry. 2013; **28**(5): 315–26.
17. **Craig TK, Garety P, Power P, Rahaman N, Colbert S, Fornells-Ambrojo M**, et al. The Lambeth Early Onset (LEO) Team: randomised controlled trial of the effectiveness of specialised care for early psychosis. BMJ. 2004; **329**(7474):14.
18. **Birchwood M.** Early intervention in psychotic relapse: cognitive approaches to detection and management. Behav Change. 1995; **12**(1):2–19.
19. **Kuipers E, Holloway F, Rabe-Hesketh S, Tennakoon L.** An RCT of early intervention in psychosis: Croydon Outreach and Assertive Support Team (COAST). Soc Psychiatry Psychiatr Epidemiol. 2004; **39**(5):358–63.
20. **McGorry PD, Nelson B, Amminger GP, Bechdolf A, Francey SM, Berger G**, et al. Intervention in individuals at ultra-high risk for psychosis: a review and future directions. J Clin Psychiatry 2009; **70**(9):1206.

21. **Bertelsen, M.**, et al., Five-year follow-up of a randomized multicenter trial of intensive early intervention vs standard treatment for patients with a first episode of psychotic illness: the OPUS trial. Arch Gen Psychiatry. 2008; **65**(7):762–71.
22. **Bird, V.**, et al., Early intervention services, cognitive–behavioural therapy and family intervention in early psychosis: systematic review. Br J Psychiatry. 2010; **197**(5):350–6.
23. **Perera G, Broadbent M, Callard F, Chang C-K, Downs J, Dutta R**, et al. Cohort profile of the South London and Maudsley NHS Foundation Trust Biomedical Research Centre (SLaM BRC) case register: current status and recent enhancement of an electronic mental health record-derived data resource. BMJ Open. 2016; **6**(3):e008721.
24. **Codd E.** A relational model of data for large shared data banks. 1970. MD Comput. 1998; **15**(3):162–6.
25. **Jablensky A, Sartorius N, Ernberg G, Anker M, Korten A, Cooper JE**, et al. Schizophrenia: manifestations, incidence and course in different cultures. A World Health Organization ten-country study. Psychol Med Monogr Suppl. 1992; **20**:1–97.
26. **Office for National Statistics (ONS)**. Ethnic group statistics: a guide for collection and classification of ethnicity data. 2003; ONS.
27. **Mallett R.** MRC Sociodemographic Schedule. Section of Social Psychiatry, Institute of Psychiatry; 1997.
28. **World Health Organization (WHO)**. Personal and Psychiatric History Schedule. Geneva: WHO; 1996.
29. StataCorp. Stata Statistical Software: Release 12. College Station, TX: StataCorp LP; 2011.
30. **Mann F, Fisher HL, Major B, Lawrence J, Tapfumaneyi A, Joyce J**, et al. Ethnic variations in compulsory detention and hospital admission for psychosis across four UK Early Intervention Services. BMC Psychiatry. 2014; **14**(1):256.
31. **Singh SP, Grange T.** Measuring pathways to care in first-episode psychosis: a systematic review. Schizophr Res. 2006; **81**(1):75–82.
32. **Mulder CL, Koopmans GT, Selten JP.** Emergency psychiatry, compulsory admissions and clinical presentation among immigrants to the Netherlands. Br J Psychiatry. 2006; **188**:386–91.
33. **Anderson K, Flora N, Archie S, Morgan C, McKenzie K**, et al. A meta-analysis of ethnic differences in pathways to care at the first episode of psychosis. Acta Psychiatr Scand. 2014; **130**(4):257–65.
34. **Bhui K, Stansfeld S, Hull S, Priebe S, Mole F, Feder G**, et al. Ethnic variations in pathways to and use of specialist mental health services in the UK systematic review. Br J Psychiatry. 2003; **182**(2):105–16.
35. **Sass B, Bhui K, Moffat J, Mckenzie K.** Enhancing pathways to care for black and minority ethnic populations: a systematic review. Int Rev Psychiatry. 2009; **21**(5):430–8.
36. **National Institute for Health and Care Excellence (NICE)**. Psychosis and schizophrenia in adults. 2015. Available from: https://www.nice.org.uk/guidance/qs80.
37. **Birchwood M, Connor C, Lester H, Patterson P, Freemantle N, Marshall M**, et al. Reducing duration of untreated psychosis: care pathways to early intervention in psychosis services. Br J Psychiatry. 2013; **203**(1):58–64.

Chapter 8

Early intervention for psychosis

Perspective after 15 years of development

Eric Y.H. Chen, Sherry Kit-wa Chan, Wing-chung Chang, Christy Lai-ming Hui, Edwin Ho-ming Lee, Tak-lam Lo, Catherine Shiu-yin Chong, Wai-song Yeung, Roger Man-kin Ng, Eric Fuk-chi Cheung, Dicky Wai-sau Chung, and Lap-tak Poon

Introduction

Early intervention (EI) for psychosis has been an important paradigm for mental health service development in the past two decades [1]. The paradigm has resulted in many specialized programmes worldwide, aimed at providing timely care for people with psychotic disorders [2, 3]. Over this period, programme development has been frequently coupled with outcome research. This has enabled a nuanced gathering of knowledge of the various aspects of the early psychosis paradigm. It is particularly important to consider the results of EI programmes in real-life situations, in order that successful experiences may be disseminated and unsuccessful efforts noted [4]. In this chapter, we use a detailed real-life example of early intervention for psychosis in Hong Kong to facilitate consideration of a broad range of perspectives. The example in Hong Kong is particularly relevant because of the cultural (modern metropolitan) background of East Asia—the comprehensive service system for a population of 7.5 million [5].

The interaction of service development with research initiatives generated an approach that was guided by empirical data addressing different key components of the early intervention methodology:

1. Early detection: the objective is to shorten the delays in help-seeking and treatment for psychotic disorders.

2. Critical period outcome: the objective is to improve outcome in the critical period by specialized focused intervention, in the hope that this outcome could be carried over to the long term.
3. Indicated prevention: the objective is to identify subjects at increased risk of developing psychosis and to provide preventative intervention that could reduce the full-blown development of psychosis (transitions). This work is still in early development in Hong Kong.

The Hong Kong Early Psychosis Programme (EASY Programme)

The cultural and societal context in Hong Kong

Hong Kong had a population of approximately 7.5 million in 2016. As a major metropolitan area in East Asia, with a heritage of predominantly Chinese culture, it has a long history of being a hub of East–West cultural exchange. However, despite the general affluence of the city, resources dedicated to mental healthcare have not been comparable with the expectation. The number of psychiatrists is 4 per 100,000 population, compared to 15–20 per 100,000 in OECD (Organisation for Economic Co-operation and Development) countries [6]. Trained mental health professionals such as nurses, social workers, clinical psychologists, and occupational therapists, are likewise in short supply [7]. As a result, services are centred around inpatient units and busy outpatient clinics. In the outpatient clinic, patients have consultation sessions averaging five minutes, once every three to four months [8]. Not surprisingly, apart from the main symptoms and medication, other needs and issues are difficult to address. This situation is not unusual amongst neighbouring, likewise affluent, East Asian populations, such as those of China, Taiwan, Singapore, Korea, and Japan.

At the turn of the millennium, before the development of the city's early psychosis service, people with a psychotic disorder on average suffered from psychotic symptoms for 1.5 years before receiving effective treatment [9]. First psychotic episodes are usually treated in inpatient settings, often precipitated by a crisis that may require compulsory hospitalization. Treatment focuses on the control of positive symptoms with medications. However, after discharge, negative symptoms increase. Suicide occurs at an alarming rate of over 3 per cent during the first three years of a first-episode cohort [10–12].

The Hong Kong Early Psychosis Programme (EASY Programme) was initiated in 2001. Programme resources were entirely in terms of manpower. Four teams were established, to each cover a defined catchment area of around 1.5–1.8 million residents. Each of the teams had two psychiatrists and three nurses, and one clinical psychologist was shared between the teams. It was recognized that the manpower would not be sufficient to cover all cases of first-onset psychosis. The programme then elected to focus on younger patients (with onset before 25 years), as outcomes are generally estimated to be more unfavourable in this group. The launching of a territory-wide service limited the opportunity for the direct use of randomized controlled study methodology in outcome evaluation.

Early detection

The DUP data for Hong Kong provided the basis for our early detection strategy. Our data [9] suggested that the DUP did not follow a normal distribution. About a third of patients present within one month, a half within six months, and two thirds within a year [5] (Fig. 8.1).

Factors related to long DUP were insidious illness onset and lack of family experience of psychosis; families with another member suffering from psychosis had shorter DUP. These two factors interacted with one another [13] (Fig.

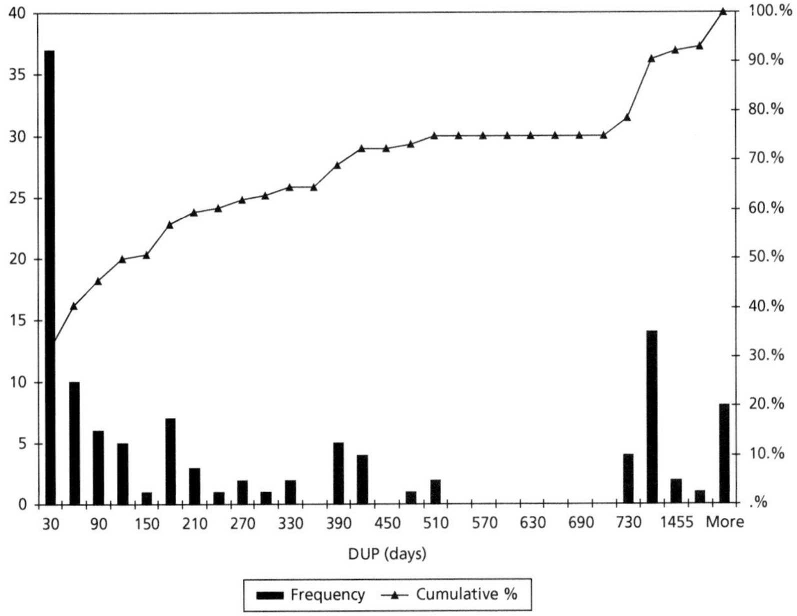

Fig. 8.1 Distribution and cumulative frequencies of duration of untreated psychosis (DUP) in Hong Kong.

Reprinted from *Early Psychosis Intervention: A Culturally Adaptive Clinical Guide* (p. 18), by E. Y. H. Chen, H, Lee, G. H. K. Chan and G. H. Y. Wong (Eds.), 2013, Hong Kong University Press. Copyright 2013 by the Hong Kong University Press. Reprinted with permission.

8.2). Living alone (though uncommon in Hong Kong due to high accommodation costs), as well as lower educational levels, were marginally significant factors [13].

The importance of family experience suggests that improving knowledge could be strategically important in reducing DUP. To improve the knowledge of potential carers before the patient presents to the health service requires a population-based approach. Media strategies focus on brief and clear messages about the nature of psychotic symptoms, the need to seek help, as well as the provision of a hot-line telephone number. To facilitate communication with the public about psychotic symptoms, it was recognized that the Chinese translation of 'psychosis' (literally meaning 'severe mental illness') was not helpful [5]. A new term was adopted, meaning 'dysregulations in thinking and perception' [14]. It is noteworthy that we adopted this term for 'psychosis' for public communication, rather than changing the official administrative Chinese term for schizophrenia [15, 16]. This strategy is significant in that it allows the new terms for psychosis to be used concurrently with the old term for schizophrenia. This parallel availability of terms enables the public and the media to selectively choose which term to use in a specific context. Generally, the media in Hong Kong have elected to use the new term in more positive and educational contexts, while the old term for schizophrenia is used in contexts with potentially

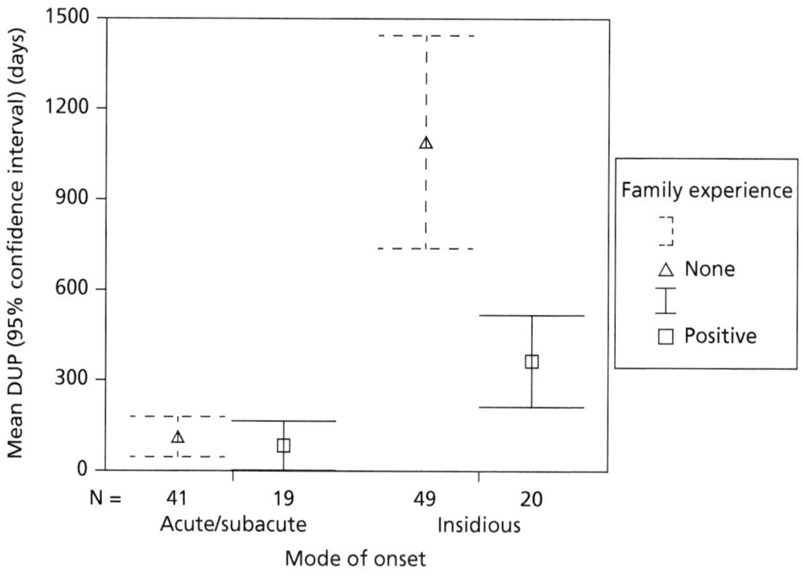

Fig. 8.2 Interaction between family experience and mode of onset in affecting duration of untreated psychosis (DUP).

negative connotations, such as incidents involving violence. It was observed that this flexibility has reduced association with the new term in a negative event which was widely reported in the city [17].

The overall impact of early detection efforts on DUP has been observed through structured DUP assessment data for 2000 to 2010 [18]. The data showed a significant reduction in DUP in the period in the adult patient population (over 25 years of age) (from median 180 days to 93 days, U=12906, p=0.01) but not in the youth population (aged 15 to 25) (from median 120 days to 90 days, U=2026, p=0.63). The reduction in DUP was particularly notable for those with a lack of family experience of psychosis (from median 285 days to 108.5 days, U=5776, p=0.01) and, in particular, for those with insidious illness onset (from median 745 days to 238 days, U=1949, p=0.01) (i.e. in groups where the DUP was longest at baseline). We established that in Hong Kong it was possible to reduce DUP for subgroups with a longer DUP (around six months), but for groups with a shorter initial DUP (around three months), further reduction was challenging.

A wide range of DUP has been reported from different locations. Only a small number of reports address the change of DUP as a result of intervention, with mixed results. This is hardly surprising as DUP is expected to be sensitive to population-specific factors such as stigma and service delivery systems. Early detection efforts also vary substantially in terms of strategy, means, and penetration. It seems important that for a particular population, early detection efforts are guided by local data. Ongoing monitoring of DUP data can also be a pragmatic measure for public services that are likely to be engaging the majority of psychosis patients in the population.

The effects of phase-specific intervention

Once a patient has been diagnosed as suffering from a psychotic disorder, intervention is initiated and delivered by a multidisciplinary team specializing in early psychosis. Case management is a core component of the intervention. In real life, manpower is limited and the average caseload is high (i.e. 80, compared to 20–30 in programmes in other countries). Case management follows a protocol [5] and consists of psychoeducation, engagement, monitoring, and counselling components [3] (Fig. 8.3). During the period between 2001 and 2011, EASY intervention was provided for a period of two years for first episode psychosis patients aged 15–25 years old, after which there was a step-down process of cessation of case management, and then transferred from the specialized early psychosis clinic to the general adult psychiatry clinic. Since 2011, EASY service is extended to three-year early intervention for all first episode psychosis patients aged 15–64 years.

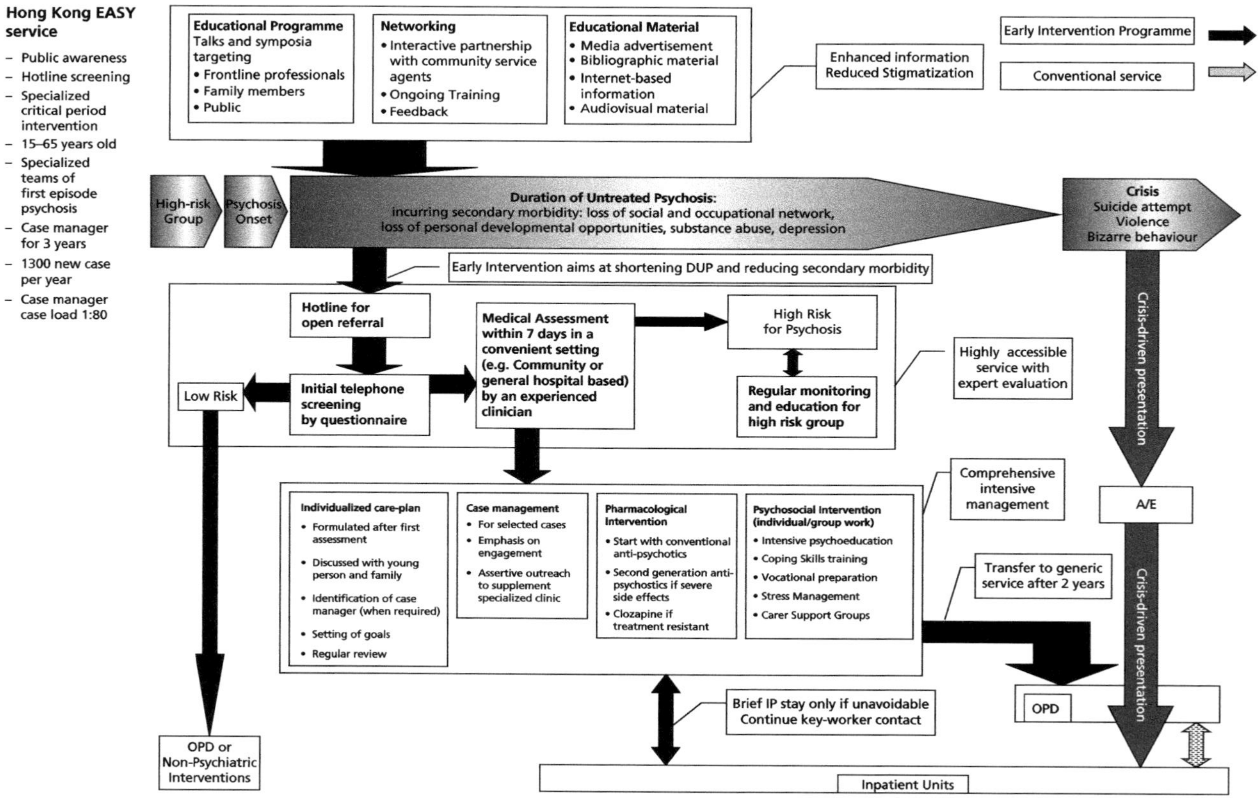

Fig. 8.3 Key components of the EASY service.

Reprinted from *Best care in early psychosis intervention: global perspectives*, T. Ehmann, G. W. MacEwan and W. G. Honer, p. 129. Copyright (2004) by Taylor and Francis Group.

Outcome studies and the critical period hypothesis

Evaluation has been carried out systematically, using patient functioning as the primary outcome variable, with suicide, psychopathology, and hospitalization as secondary outcome variables. The questions we asked of the intervention data in Hong Kong were as follows:

- Did the provision of a two-year early intervention programme make a difference to outcome?
- If the outcome is improved, can it be sustained over time (e,g, in ten years)?
- Can the early outcome be further improved by providing an additional period of intervention (e.g. whether three years of intervention is superior to two years)?
- If the additional intervention leads to an even better outcome, can it be sustained?

We approached these questions with a series of studies addressing the immediate outcome of the EASY service. We adopted a cohort study comparing outcome of patients who were diagnosed and managed just before the launch of the EASY programme (standard care) to a group of comparable patients who were managed in the EASY programme (early intervention) [19].

The results demonstrated an improvement in functioning and a reduction in hospitalization; however, the relapse rates were unchanged [19]. It is noteworthy that the improvement in functional outcome was present from the initial episode, which suggests that management of the first episode plays a crucial role in maintaining occupational functioning. One distinctive feature of the EI care was the need for inpatient treatment: previously, 90 per cent of first-episode patients required this; now, 50% of patients could avoid it. The circumvention of inpatient treatment may have important consequences for functional outcome, as many patients could stand to lose their jobs during a period of such treatment. It is also important to note that for this group of younger patients, the DUP was not significantly changed. This provided a unique opportunity to specifically confirm the effects of intervention (rather than early detection), without having to disentangle potential contributions from DUP shortening.

After demonstrating a positive effect of early intervention, we next asked whether this effect can be maintained over a longer period, after ceasing input from the EASY programme. To address this, we conducted a ten-year follow-up study [20]. The results suggest that improvements in functioning, reduction in hospital admissions, and suicide reduction were maintained, even after the cessation of direct EASY input. The significant reduction in suicide is particularly noteworthy. These data provided support for the rationale for critical period intervention.

When we then studied the effects of an additional year of intervention, it was possible to adopt a RCT (randomized controlled trial) design. We randomized people who already had had two years of early intervention into a group that received one more year of intervention, as well as a control group that received standard care [21] (Fig. 8.4). The results showed that an additional year of early intervention resulted in further improvements in functioning, while the control group did not make further progress and maintained the previous level of functioning [21]. These findings suggest that after two years of intervention there is still room for further improvement in functioning, which can be attained by providing an additional year of intervention. However, subsequent follow-up studies revealed that this further improvement was not sustained [W.C. Chang, personal communication, 14 January 2017].

A model of intervention effectiveness

Using real-life intervention data from Hong Kong, the impact of early intervention in a relatively low-resource setting can be summarized in Fig. 8.5 and as follows:

- A two-year basic early intervention programme led to the immediate outcome of improved occupational functioning and reduced hospitalization. This was achieved without significant changes in DUP.
- These effects could be sustained beyond the two-year direct intervention period. Reduction in hospitalization and suicide rates, as well as improvement in functioning, were observable in ten-year follow-up. Improvements were not only observed in the initial critical period years but also in the subsequent years.
- Improvement in functional outcome could be further enhanced by the provision of an additional year of intervention (three years versus two years).
- However, the enhancement attributable to an additional year of intervention was not sustained.

How do we reconcile the observations that (1) basic intervention effects (year 1–2) were sustainable while (2) additional intervention effects (year 3) were not? The nature of intervention was similar in both cases. What differed was (i) the timing of the intervention—year 1 and year 2 in the case of basic intervention, compared to year 3 in the case of additional intervention; (ii) the patients recruited in the study were selected because they had made relatively less progress after already receiving two years of intervention; (iii) background

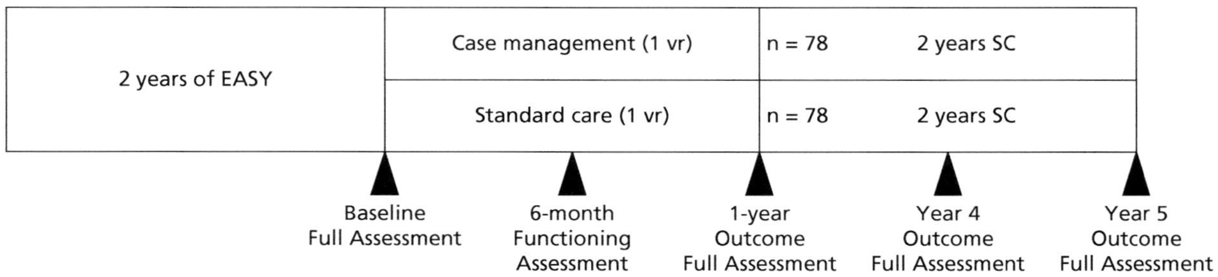

Fig. 8.4 Randomized controlled trial (RCT) design for investigating effects of additional intervention time.

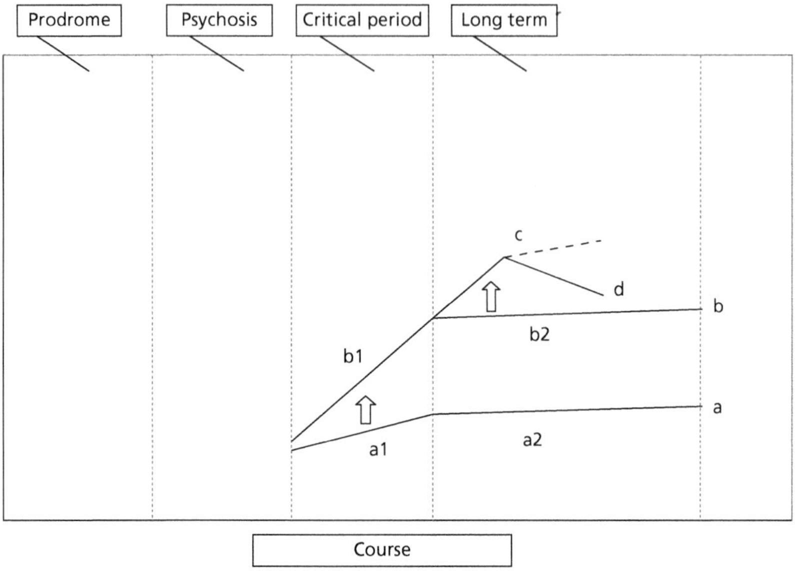

Fig. 8.5 Schematic summary of early intervention (EI) effects on functional outcomes: (a) standard care before EI, showing some improvements in functioning over time; (b) functional outcome with basic two-year EI—b1 shows that improvement is observed during intervention period (two years), b2 shows that improved outcome is sustained after EI is withdrawn; (c) indicates that further intervention period (year 3) leads to further outcome improvements; (d) further improvement is more difficult to sustain after EI has ceased.

mental health service development and the availability of other services for the control group was lower for the basic intervention study compared with the additional intervention study; thus, there was an increased possibility of catch up in the control group.

It is possible to summarize the findings and interpretation of the series of interventions with a model on intervention effects. In this model, we postulate that intervention effect and its maintenance is related to the intensity of intervention (higher, stronger), the timing of intervention (earlier, better), and the level of existing functioning (the higher, the more difficult to further improve). This data provides some rationale for prioritization on the timing and duration of phase-specific intervention in circumstances where there is resource limitation.

$$\frac{\text{F(Timing)(Intensity)}}{\text{(Functional Level)}} = \text{Momentum}$$

The Hong Kong early intervention outcome data has adopted conventional measurements of quantitative data, allowing alignment with evidence-based medicine. It is important also to recognize that quantitative methods have limitations in early psychosis service development. A conventional quantitative approach, using group comparison, may inhibit the development of a more personalized approach to service design. It may also restrict the view on some important aspects of early psychosis work, such as a positive service culture and an emphasis on hope.

Conclusions: a new integrative experiential-neuroscientific approach

Recent advances in neuroscience have enhanced our understanding about the extent to which the brain is modifiable in response to different environmental and psychosocial inputs, including actions initiated by the subjects [22–25]. Patients' understanding of the illness and their individual roles should take these findings into consideration. This emerging paradigm no longer places the person, in a deterministic manner, as just a passive downstream consequence of brain processes, but supports a view that is far more interactive and bi-directional, in that one's choices and actions can have effects on brain structure and processes [26–28]. It is important that this new perspective be emphasized in public awareness and patient education messages, so that a more positive and hopeful representation of the illness can be embraced.

In early psychosis, intervention is characterized by the subjective nature of the illness, its aetiology, and its course, in which the outcome is unknown to both the patient and the clinician, and the disease continues to unfold over a number of years [29]. The emphasis on hope is implicit, in the recognition that at least for a proportion of patients, the course of the illness can be favourable. In truly collaborative casework, the possibility of positive expectation can act to minimize negative self-fulfilling prophecy, while the unfolding of disappointments can also be supported in an ongoing, prepared manner [5, 30, 31]. This approach sustains a measured optimism which can facilitate the best possible outcome. In those whose outcome is less favourable, there is the possibility of a supported transition from the high initial expectation to the realities of a more modest long-term outcome without a sense of dejection. Within this framework, even a less favourable outcome can be embraced and handled with a more positive mindset, dovetailing with modern concepts of recovery [32].

Summary

This chapter provides a comprehensive review of some of the key issues in early intervention for psychosis using the example of a population-based service in Hong Kong, for which a full range of data is available. It focuses on the optimal detection and management of first-episode psychosis, and shows that even in a low-resource setting, significant improvements in functioning can be achieved, with reduced hospitalization admissions and reduced suicide rates. A long-term follow-up study observed that these effects are sustainable. Further improvements can be attained by providing a longer period of intervention to those that respond less favourably. However, these enhancements prove more difficult to sustain. Together, these suggest a possible dose effect on the impact and sustainability of early intervention for psychosis. Future work should aim to clarify the role of increased intervention resources (e.g. manpower) and a more defined specific programme (e.g. coaching, exercise, cognitive interventions). More work is also required to investigate the culture of early psychosis services, as well as how the personalized needs of individual patients can be met.

References

1. **McGorry PD, Killackey E, Yung A.** Early intervention in psychosis: concepts, evidence and future directions. World Psychiatry. 2008; **7**(3):148–56.
2. **Edwards J, McGorry PD.** Implementing early intervention in psychosis: a guide to establishing early psychosis services. London: Martin Dunitz; 2002. p. xv, 186.
3. **Ehmann T, MacEwan GW, Honer WG.** Best care in early psychosis intervention: global perspectives. London, New York: Taylor & Francis; 2004.
4. **Chen EYH, Wong GHY, Lam MML, Chiu CPY, Hui CLM.** Real-world implementation of early intervention in psychosis: resources, funding models and evidence-based practice. World Psychiatry. 2008; **7**(3):163–4.
5. **Chen EY-h, Lee H, Chan GH-k, Wong GH-y,** editors. Early psychosis intervention: a culturally adaptive clinical guide. Hong Kong: Hong Kong University Press; 2013.
6. **Organisation for Economic Co-operation and Development (OECD).** OECD reviews of health care quality. Raising standards. Paris: OECD; 2012.
7. **Chan WC, Lam LCW, Chen EYH.** Hong Kong: recent development of mental health services. Adv Psychiatr Treat. 2015; **21**(1):71–2.
8. **Hui CLM, Wong GHY, Lam CYK, Chow PPL, Chen EYH.** Patient-clinician communication and needs identification for outpatients with schizophrenia in Hong Kong: potential role of the 2-COM instrument. Hong Kong J Psychiatry. 2008; **18**:69–75.
9. **Chen EY, Dunn EL, Miao MY, Yeung WS, Wong CK, Chan WF,** et al. The impact of family experience on the duration of untreated psychosis (DUP) in Hong Kong. Soc Psychiatry Psychiatr Epidemiol. 2005; **40**(5):350–6.

10. **Chang WC, Hui CL, Tang JY, Wong GH, Chan SK, Lee EH**, et al. Impacts of duration of untreated psychosis on cognition and negative symptoms in first-episode schizophrenia: a 3-year prospective follow-up study. Psychol Med. 2013; **43**(9):1883–93.
11. **Chiu CPY, Tang JYM, Chen EYH, Hui CLM, Law CW, Yew C**, et al. Outcome of an Early Intervention Programme for Psychosis (EASY). Early Interv Psychiatry. 2008; **2**:A112.
12. **Wong G, Hui C, Chiu C, Lam M, Chung D, Tso S**, et al. Early detection and intervention of psychosis in Hong Kong: experience of a population-based intervention programme. Clin Neuropsychiatry. 2008; **5**(6):286–9.
13. **Chen EY, Hui CL, Dunn EL, Miao MY, Yeung WS, Wong CK**, et al. A prospective 3-year longitudinal study of cognitive predictors of relapse in first-episode schizophrenic patients. Schizophr Res. 2005; **77**(1):99–104.
14. **Chiu CP, Lam MM, Chan SK, Chung DW, Hung SF, Tang JY**, et al. Naming psychosis: the Hong Kong experience. Early Interv Psychiatry. 2010; **4**(4):270–4.
15. **Lee YS, Kim JJ, Kwon JS.** Renaming schizophrenia in South Korea. Lancet. 2013; **382**(9893):683–4.
16. **Sato M.** Renaming schizophrenia: a Japanese perspective. World Psychiatry. 2006; **5**(1):53–5.
17. **Tam W, Tang JY, Chan SK, Hui CL, Wong GH, Lam MM**, et al. Public attitudes toward psychosis following a tragic violent incident in Hong Kong. Early Interv Psychiatry. 2010; **4**(Suppl s1):77.
18. **Chan SK, Chau EH, Hui CL, Chang WC, Lee EH, Chen EY.** Long term effect of early intervention service on duration of untreated psychosis in youth and adult population in Hong Kong. Early Interv Psychiatry. 2018; **12**(3):331–8
19. **Chen EY, Tang JY, Hui CL, Chiu CP, Lam MM, Law CW**, et al. Three-year outcome of phase-specific early intervention for first-episode psychosis: a cohort study in Hong Kong. Early Interv Psychiatry. 2011; **5**(4):315–23.
20. **Chan SK, So HC, Hui CL, Chang WC, Lee EH, Chung DW**, et al. 10-year outcome study of an early intervention program for psychosis compared with standard care service. Psychol Med. 2015; **45**(6):1181–93.
21. **Chang WC, Chan GH, Jim OT, Lau ES, Hui CL, Chan SK**, et al. Optimal duration of an early intervention programme for first-episode psychosis: randomised controlled trial. Br J Psychiatry. 2015; **206**(6):492–500.
22. **Haddad L, Schafer A, Streit F, Lederbogen F, Grimm O, Wust S**, et al. Brain structure correlates of urban upbringing, an environmental risk factor for schizophrenia. Schizophr Bull. 2015; **41**(1):115–22.
23. **Lee SW, Yoo JH, Kim KW, Lee JS, Kim D, Park H**, et al. Aberrant function of frontoamygdala circuits in adolescents with previous verbal abuse experiences. Neuropsychologia. 2015; **79**:76–85.
24. **Malchow B, Keeser D, Keller K, Hasan A, Rauchmann BS, Kimura H**, et al. Effects of endurance training on brain structures in chronic schizophrenia patients and healthy controls. Schizophr Res. 2016; **173**(3):182–91.
25. **Puetz VB, Parker D, Kohn N, Dahmen B, Verma R, Konrad K.** Altered brain network integrity after childhood maltreatment: a structural connectomic DTI-study. Hum Brain Mapp. 2017; **38**(2):855–68.

26. **Power JD, Schlaggar BL.** Neural plasticity across the lifespan. Wiley Interdiscip Rev Dev Biol. 2017; **6**(1).
27. **Richmond S, Johnson KA, Seal ML, Allen NB, Whittle S.** Development of brain networks and relevance of environmental and genetic factors: a systematic review. Neurosci Biobehav Rev. 2016; **71**:215–39.
28. **Sale A, Berardi N, Maffei L.** Environment and brain plasticity: towards an endogenous pharmacotherapy. Physiol Rev. 2014; **94**(1):189–234.
29. **Good BJ.** Medicine, rationality and experience: an anthropological perspective. Cambridge: Cambridge University Press; 1993.
30. **Horan WP, Kern RS, Shokat-Fadai K, Sergi MJ, Wynn JK, Green MF.** Social cognitive skills training in schizophrenia: an initial efficacy study of stabilized outpatients. Schizophr Res. 2009; **107**(1):47–54.
31. **Thornicroft G, Susser E.** Evidence-based psychotherapeutic interventions in the community care of schizophrenia. The British journal of psychiatry: the journal of mental science. 2001;**178**(1):2–4.
32. **Davidson L, O'Connell MJ, Tondora J, Lawless M, Evans AC.** Recovery in serious mental illness: A new wine or just a new bottle? Prof Psychol-Res Pr. 2005;**36**(5):480–7.

Chapter 9

Experiences and lessons from the Singapore Early Psychosis Intervention Programme

Swapna K. Verma, Poon Lye Yin, Helen Lee, and Chong Siow Ann

Background

Singapore is a small city state in South-east Asia and has a population of about 5.2 million, of which 3.8 million are Singaporean citizens or permanent residents. Of these, approximately 74 per cent are of Chinese descent, 13 per cent are Malay, and 9 per cent are Indian [1]. The only state mental hospital in Singapore is the Institute of Mental Health (IMH). It is a 2,000-bed acute tertiary psychiatric hospital that offers a comprehensive range of psychiatric, rehabilitative, and counselling services for people of all ages. In the 1980s, the IMH worked towards changing its image of one of a custodial institution to a centre offering therapeutic activities in the community. From the 1980s to the early 2000s, psychiatric units were set up in general hospitals and liaison medicine was encouraged. The private sector also emerged in the early 1970s, providing a more conducive inpatient and outpatient environment and personable service at a higher cost [2]. In Singapore, primary healthcare is provided by government polyclinics and private general medical practitioner clinics. There is no patient list system, and patients have the freedom of selecting any doctor they wish to see. Patients therefore have direct and easy access to specialists. A recent study categorized Singapore as a 'low' primary care country, particularly in relation to areas such as specialist care, accessibility of care, and care continuity [3].

The IMH remains the single largest tertiary care facility in Singapore, where the majority of the patients with serious mental illnesses such as schizophrenia and bipolar disorder receive their treatment. A study conducted at the IMH in the year 2000, that looked at the duration of untreated psychosis (DUP) and pathways to care in Singapore, found that the mean DUP was 32.6 months (SD=59.8), with a median of 12 months [4]. Despite the relatively easy access to healthcare in Singapore, the DUP of our patients was relatively long, and this appeared to be largely due to 'patient delay'(i.e. the time between onset of symptoms and help-seeking). Other than the lack of insight into their condition, the long delay in seeking help may have been due to certain cultural factors operating in Singapore society and the attribution of other explanations for the psychotic symptoms. The concept of 'face' is particularly prevalent among the Chinese. The abnormal behaviour of a psychotic individual is seen as bringing shame and/or embarrassment to the family and, as a 'face-saving' strategy, family members often resort to denying or disguising the manifestation of mental illness. Another interesting finding was that 24 per cent of patients had sought consultation with a traditional healer prior to consulting a psychiatrist, suggesting that beliefs in supernatural causes of mental disorders were widely held and that traditional sources of help for such health issues, such as spiritual healers, were preferred to Western-trained physicians.

The Early Psychosis Intervention Programme: a new model of care

The alarmingly long DUP and its possible consequences, and the preference for traditional and spiritual healers for psychotic disorders (which called into question the appropriateness of care), were the impetus for establishing the Early Psychosis Intervention Programme (EPIP). The programme was initiated in April 2001 under the auspices of the Health Services Development Programme of the Singapore Ministry of Health [5]. The EPIP set out to do the following:

- Raise awareness of the early signs and symptoms of psychosis, and reduce the stigma associated with it.
- Establish strong links with primary healthcare providers and collaborate in the detection, referral, and management of those with psychosis.
- Improve the outcome and quality of life of those with psychosis, and reduce the burden of care for their families.

Outreach

We have used a multi-pronged approach to educate the public which has included public forums, radio and television interviews, a television documentary drama on psychosis, press releases, a book on psychosis aimed at the general public, posters displayed at train stations, art exhibitions, public events that enlisted the help of local celebrities, a website (www.epip.org.sg), and a hotline telephone service.

Establishing collaborations

Initiatives were launched with the aim of educating, networking, and collaborating with primary healthcare providers (private general practitioners (GPs) and polyclinic doctors, counsellors from the various institutes of higher learning, social and welfare services, and traditional Chinese medicine (TCM) practitioners). We have also built close collaboration with the Singapore Armed Forces, as Singapore has a large standing conscript army and all Singaporean males are required to do two years of National Service upon turning 18 years of age. In addition, to help in the reintegration of our patients back into the community, we established the EPIP-GP Partnership Programme which involves GPs in the ongoing management of stable patients in the community.

A patient-centred clinical service

We aimed to create a comprehensive, integrated, multidisciplinary, and patient-centred programme. Patients are accepted into EPIP if they are aged between 16 and 40 years and present with first-episode psychosis. Exclusion criteria are as follows:

1. organic psychosis, including drug- and alcohol-induced psychosis;
2. established treatment resistance (not resolved even after six months of adequate treatment with two trials of optimal-dosage antipsychotic medication);
3. current remand or complex forensic cases; and
4. learning disability (based on IQ or functional assessment).

Patients are typically followed up for a period of three years before they are transferred to secondary-level community-based care.

We have a multidisciplinary team that is competent, culturally sensitive, and skilled in providing phase-specific care. We made case management a core competency and have ensured that the case managers maintain their edge through continuous training and supervision. We started 'Club EPIP', with a club-like environment where patients are able to receive ongoing support, to participate in rehabilitative programmes that prepare them to return to school or work, and to socialize and build meaningful relationships with others. Gradually, but surely, the team has adapted to a more strengths-based, recovery-focused model of care underpinned by psychosocial interventions that could truly empower our patients and their families.

Families play a critical role in the recovery of our patients, since the majority of patients (96.3 per cent) continue to live with them [6]. Hence, EPIP has a strong focus on helping families, starting out with family psychoeducation workshops “and evolving into”, multifamily and individual family therapies, as well as support offered by family peer specialists. The EPIP peer support programme plays a significant role in our patients’ care. In fact, our experience has shown us that peer support is valuable as an adjunct to the mainstay psychosocial support of case managers. The peer support specialist shares his or her recovery story, and instils hope in those still recovering and coping with their psychotic illness.

In February 2016, the EPIP opened a 20-bed inpatient unit for the acute treatment of young people with first-episode psychosis. Designed to facilitate therapeutic work and recovery, it boasts of features such as an open pantry, a night lounge, and an outdoor garden. While introducing new processes and facilities in the ward, the multidisciplinary care team, along with recovered patients, engaged in various quality-improvement discussions to proactively ensure that workflow and ward designs were safe for clients and staff, and promoted support and recovery.

Systematic evaluation and research

We felt that it was vital to set up a structured system of evaluating our patients—at first contact and, subsequently, at regular intervals—using structured rating instruments. Patients are evaluated on the severity of symptoms, the presence of side-effects, overall functioning, quality of life, and service satisfaction. The resultant database has been a rich source of information that has helped us in monitoring the quality and outcomes of our service, that has made us accountable to our stakeholders and funders, and has generated data for various research studies. The emerging key outcomes have been:

1. *Reduction in DUP*: The median duration of untreated psychosis fell from twelve months to four months in the two years following the start of the programme. In the first year of the programme, 9.1 per cent of clients were referred from the primary healthcare sector; this had climbed to 22.6 per cent by the end of the second year. There was also a 10.7 per cent increase in the proportion of self and family referrals ($p=0.04$), and a 15.2 per cent fall in the proportion of police referrals ($p=0.001$) which indicated that there were fewer cases that were brought by the police because of a crisis—possibly because of earlier help-seeking behaviour [7].
2. *Remission*: At the end of a two-year follow-up, 54.1 per cent of our 1,125 patients had achieved symptomatic remission, based on the criteria proposed by the Schizophrenia Working Group; 58.4 per cent had achieved significant functional remission, based on a priori defined criteria; and 29.4 per cent met criteria for both symptomatic and functional remission [8].

3. *Service engagement*: 86 per cent of our 775 patients remained engaged with our service, either through face-to-face contact or telephone contact, during a two-year follow-up [9].
4. *Suicide rates*: In a study among 1,397 of our patients, prevalence of suicide in the first two years of the service was found to be 1.9 per cent [13], which was close to the 1 per cent bench mark recommended by the World Health Organization (WHO) Declaration on Early Psychosis [10].

The National Mental Health Blueprint: the next phase

In April 2007, the EPIP came under Singapore's first National Mental Health Blueprint. Drawn up by the Ministry of Health (MOH), together with stakeholders, the Blueprint aimed to promote mental health and, where possible, prevent the development of mental health disorders as well as reduce their impact. The Blueprint had four main thrusts: mental health promotion, integrated mental healthcare, developing manpower, and research and evaluation. It injected some additional funds and gave us an opportunity to push the envelope, moving into 'indicated prevention' and youth mental health.

Indicated prevention: Support for Wellness Achievement Programme

The Support for Wellness Achievement Programme (SWAP) was started in April 2008 to provide a treatment service for help-seeking individuals between the ages of 16–30 years who were experiencing an at-risk mental state (ARMS). Phillips et al. [11] have defined an operational set of clinical features that can be used to identify individuals presenting with an ARMS, and this criterion has been adopted by SWAP. Individuals are deemed to have an ARMS if they fulfil the criteria for any of the following three groups, in addition to a decline in functioning during the preceding year:

- *Vulnerability group*: individuals with a family history of a psychotic disorder in a first-degree relative, or a diagnosis of schizotypal personality disorder.
- *Attenuated symptom group*: individuals with attenuated or low-grade psychotic symptoms that are deemed to be of subthreshold frequency or intensity.
- *Brief limited intermittent psychotic symptoms (BLIPS) group*: individuals who have experienced a frank psychotic episode that resolved spontaneously within a week.

SWAP also uses a multidisciplinary team approach, and management is based on a biopsychosocial model of care. Psychotropic medication is prescribed for any existing co-morbid mental disorders, but antipsychotic medication is not routinely prescribed for individuals with an ARMS unless they are extremely distressed by attenuated symptoms or specifically request it, and where the attending SWAP psychiatrist thinks it is clinically justified [12].

Moving forward into youth mental health: Community Health Assessment Team

Not all individuals who have a mental health problem may fulfil a diagnosis of a mental disorder, but the distress experienced can be both frightening and traumatic. Yet, the number of individuals coming forth to seek help has been low: the Singapore Mental Health Study [13] identified that common mental illnesses develop early in life, and of those individuals with a mental health condition, only 31.8 per cent sought help [14]. In April 2009, under the National Mental Health Blueprint, the EPIP expanded the scope of its services to include youth mental health promotion by setting up the Community Health Assessment Team (CHAT), primarily targeting young persons aged between 16 and 30 years old. The core objectives of CHAT are to raise awareness of youth mental health concerns and improve accessibility to mental health resources by reducing the barrier to entry to specialist services. CHAT's key unique offering, and the lynchpin of the service, is a free, confidential, and non-stigmatizing mental health assessment for youths experiencing mental health issues [15]. The assessment is done in a youth-friendly, shop-front facility called the CHAT hub. Young people who come forward for assessments are not registered with any hospital systems and at the end of the assessment, depending upon the young person's needs, he or she is either offered brief therapy at the CHAT hub or direct referrals are facilitated to the appropriate downstream support services (specialist outpatient clinics or follow-up at community or educational services) so as to ensure that timely treatment is instituted. In addition, young people who are assessed as suffering psychosis, and are at risk of developing psychosis, are then referred for follow-up with the EPIP and the SWAP, respectively.

CHAT has volunteers called CHAT ambassadors (mainly students and young working adults) who help in the outreach efforts to raise awareness about the importance of youth mental health, to encourage help-seeking, and to collaborate with CHAT in identifying service gaps and improving service delivery. CHAT serves to bridge the gap between mental health promotion and treatment, through early detection and intervention. While this model of early detection and intervention in the community is not new to healthcare, this approach in the field of mental health for young people is novel. Ultimately, CHAT aims to empower young people to take charge of their mental health.

References

1. **Department of Statistics, Republic of Singapore.** Population trends 2012. 2012 [accessed 2015 October 18] p. 3. Available from: http://costofhealthyliving.com/wp-content/uploads/2013/11/population2012.pdf.
2. **Ng BY, Chee KT.** A brief history of psychiatry in Singapore. Int Rev Psychiatry. 2006; **18**:335–61.
3. **Khoo HS, Lim YW, Vrijhoef HJ.** Primary healthcare system and practice characteristics in Singapore. Asia Pac Fam Med. 2014; **13**:8.
4. **Chong SA, Mythily S, Lum A, Chan YH, McGorry P.** Determinants of duration of untreated psychosis and the pathway to care in Singapore. Int J Soc Psychiatry. 2005; **51**(1):55–62.
5. **Chong SA, Verma SK, Lee C.** Psychosis—everyone's concern: the Early Psychosis Intervention Programme (EPIP) in Singapore. Singapore Fam Physician. 2001; **27**(1–2):49–52.
6. **Chesney E, Abdin E, Poon LY, Subramaniam M, Verma S.** Pathways to care for patients with first-episode psychosis in Singapore. J Nerv Ment Dis. 2016; **204**(4):291–7.
7. **Chong SA, Mythily S, Verma S.** Reducing the duration of untreated psychosis and changing help-seeking behaviour in Singapore. Soc Psychiatry Psychiatr Epidemiol. 2005; **40**(8):619–21.
8. **Verma S, Subramaniam M, Abdin E, Poon LY, Chong SA.** Symptomatic and functional remission in patients with first-episode psychosis. Acta Psychiatr Scand. 2012; **126**:282–9.
9. **Zheng S, Verma S, Poon LY.** Rate and predictors of service disengagement in patients with first-episode psychosis. Psychiatr Serv. 2013; **64**(8):812–15.
10. **Mitter N, Subramaniam M, Abdin E, Poon LY, Verma S.** Predictors of suicide in Asian patients with first episode psychosis. Schizophr Res. 2013; **151**(1–3):274–8.
11. **Phillips LJ, Yung AR, McGorry PD.** Identification of young people at risk of psychosis: validation of Personal Assessment and Crisis Evaluation Clinic intake criteria. Austr N Z J Psychiatry. 2000; **34**(suppl):S164–9.
12. **Tay S, Yuen PM, Lim LK, Pariyasami S, Rao S, Poon LY**, et al. Support for Wellness Achievement Programme (SWAP)—clinical and demographic characteristics of young people with at-risk mental state in Singapore. Early Interv Psychiatry. 2015; **9**(6):516–22.
13. **Vaingankar JA, Rekhi G, Subramaniam M, Abdin E, Chong SA.** Age of onset of life-time mental disorders and treatment contact. Soc Psychiatry Psychiatr Epidemiol. 2013; **48**(5):835–43.
14. **Chong SA, Abdin E, Vaingankar JA, Kwok KW, Subramaniam M.** Where do people with mental disorders in Singapore go to for help? Ann Acad Med Singapore. 2012; **41**:154–60.
15. **Poon LY, Tay E, Lee YP, Lee H, Verma S.** Making in-roads across the youth mental health landscape in Singapore: the Community Health Assessment Team (CHAT). Early Interv Psychiatry. 2016; **10**(2):171–7.

Chapter 10

Early psychosis initiative in Japan

Challenges and opportunities

Masafumi Mizuno, Naomi Inoue, Takahiro Nemoto, Naohisa Tsujino, Naoyuki Katagiri, and Tomoyuki Funatogawa

Introduction: Background of psychiatric services in Japan

Psychiatric services in Japan have been dominantly hospital-based for several decades. The total number of inpatients in Japanese psychiatric wards was about 308,000 in June 2010. While this number is relatively large, it is important to note that a large number of psychiatric care beds in Japan are utilized by long-stay chronic patients who might not be reported under the psychiatric bed category in other OECD (Organisation for Economic Co-operation and Development) countries [1]. Several nationwide surveys have found that approximately 20 to 40 per cent of inpatients could have been discharged if appropriate health and welfare services had been available. These cases are called 'social admissions' in Japan. A deficiency of social welfare services has forced these patients into hospitals. Today, the biggest task of psychiatry in Japan is still the deinstitutionalization of patients—not the early intervention.

The stigma of mental illness is deepened by images of hospitalization, prompting people suffering from mild mental disorders to avoid early intervention and inclusion in the community. Nevertheless, the Japanese mental healthcare system is slowly changing. Commitment and effort over the past decade is generating positive changes in the system: the number of psychiatric inpatient beds is decreasing, along with a reduction in the average length of stay in psychiatric hospitals; and community care and support provision is increasing. A recent revision of the fee schedule incentive is shifting care from hospitals to communities by further developing community-based comprehensive healthcare services. Given Japan's rapidly ageing population and low birth rate, a clear orientation towards prevention and pre-emptive approaches is surely necessary.

Care in the community for severe mental illness and the early stages of more severe mental illnesses, such as at-risk mental states, should be further enhanced. For individuals with mild to moderate disorders (e.g. depressive symptoms, anxiety, insomnia), medical care is typically delivered at mental health clinics in the community. In some cases, however, care is not easily accessible. The stigma of mental illness in Japan likely deters people from seeking help from facilities specializing in mental health. These attitudes result in a longer duration of untreated psychosis (DUP) and a higher suicide rate among young people, even in countries with sophisticated healthcare services, such as Japan.

Mental health clinics can provide pharmacological treatments and, depending on their capacity, some psychotherapies, such as counselling; they can also refer people to specialized mental health providers. On the other hand, family doctors and other physicians who perform primary care 'functions' in Japan cannot provide care to patients with mild and moderate mental disorders, since they do not receive education or training for the treatment of such disorders during their residency, and can only prescribe a fairly small range of pharmaceuticals (e.g. anti-anxietics, antidepressants, herbal (oriental) medicines) for mental healthcare. Actually, general or primary care physicians do not play a central role in the provision of care for patients with mild to moderate disorders.

Given this situation, spreading the concept of the importance of early intervention for mental health disorders is difficult. Studies and data regarding this situation originate from researchers who believe in the importance of early intervention in the community.

Culturally relevant help-seeking behaviours and barriers to services

Even in this adverse situation, some innovative hospitals have, through their own endeavours, attempted to make the transition to community-based psychiatry [2, 3]. Following the new trends for early intervention and because of several issues regarding mental health services, about ten years ago, the Ministry of Health, Welfare, and Labour (MHWL) in Japan started a research project into early intervention in mental health, under the Health Labour Sciences Research Grant. Data from this investigation shows that the mean DUP is 17.6 months. This data came from seven university hospitals, where patients can visit without facing excessive stigma. The DUP would likely be even longer if data from specialized psychiatric hospitals were included, especially those in rural areas where greater stigma around mental illness exists. About '10% of first-episode schizophrenia patients had already attempted suicide using a lethal means prior to their first consultation with a psychiatrist; this figure was higher than expected and suggests that a number of patients with untreated psychosis likely die as a result of suicide in Japan' [4].

Following the results, the MHWL has created a new website for young adolescents, which provides information regarding the importance of early intervention for mental illness [5]. Furthermore, the Japan Agency for Medical Research and Development (AMED) (https://research-er.jp/projects/view/965337) (with Principal Investigator, Masafumi Mizuno) has recently started a new project to develop treatment guidelines for early psychosis.

When thinking about the dissemination of early intervention for mental disorders in Japan, we must consider the culture and attitudes towards mental disorders among the Japanese people. Our own clinical experience shows that individuals with mental health problems, and their families, are often reluctant to seek help for various reasons, including a lack of knowledge with regard to the features and treatability of mental disorders, the belief that the problem should be solved by themselves, and the desire to confine the problem to close relations (without consulting professionals); although Japanese people generally accept the need for sophisticated treatment for physical problems. These obstacles may explain the long DUP and the social stigma of mental disorders in Japan. In addition, the nuclearization of families may also be affecting this delay in seeking treatment. These considerations should be further investigated.

A retrospective study of seven medical centres, across three cities (Tokyo, Toyama, and Kochi), has also been performed. In total, 150 consecutive patients (78 men) with neuroleptic-naive, first-episode schizophrenia were investigated; their DUP and demographic, clinical, and social variables were obtained from their medical charts and were analysed [6]. The median DUP was 6 months (mean, 20.3 months); 14 patients (9.3 per cent) had a DUP of more than 60 months, and 47 patients, or about one third, had a DUP of more than 24 months. No significant differences in the mean DUPs were observed among the three cities, but patients living alone had a significantly longer DUP.

Description of diagnosis and treatment available in Japan

In Japan (120 million population), there are some 100,000 clinics functioning as 'primary care' providers. Such care is typically delivered by semi-generalists/specialists—that is, physicians who leave hospital practice after an unspecified amount of time to set up as general physicians in the community. Family doctors and other physicians performing a primary care 'function' usually do not play a central role in the care of patients with mild and moderate mental disorders, including at-risk cases or those in the early stages of severe mental illness with less manifested psychiatric symptoms. Even psychiatrists in clinics, who recognize an at-risk mental state (ARMS) at an early stage, might not provide treatment according to recommended guidelines. Using case vignettes, Tsujino et al. investigated the abilities of psychiatrists in Japan to identify for ARMS [7]. Their results suggested that pharmacotherapy might be overused in prodromal cases. The concept of an ARMS/prodromal state might not yet be widely recognized among Japanese psychiatrists. Competency in treating and diagnosing mild and moderate disorders should be integrated into training for the primary care specialty.

Screening and diagnostic tools such as the Structured Interview for Prodromal Syndromes/the Scale of Prodromal Symptoms (SIPS/SOPS) [8, 9], the Comprehensive Assessment of At-Risk Mental States (CAARMS) [10], and the PRIME-screen, are all available in Japanese. However, personal resources in the field of psychiatry are limited.

In contrast, there is a very unique support system for mental health in schools in Japan. One or two Yogo teachers, who have completed a course in nursing and health education during the process of becoming a teacher, are designated and contribute to the health of students at each school, from primary to high school. The Japanese Association of Yogo Teacher Education defines a '*Yogo* teacher' as a specially licensed educator who supports children's growth and development through health education and health services based on the principles of health promotion in all educational activities at school. Such Yogo teachers are employed as full-time teachers at each school. The Yogo teacher provides health services and 'psychological first aid' to students; the students usually find the Yogo teacher's health room to be relaxing and comfortable. The health room, which does not have a classroom atmosphere, is a place where students can talk with the Yogo teacher who provides a 'listening ear' and, if necessary, refers students to the school counsellor.

School physicians or 'primary doctors' with practices located close to the school also visit the schools on occasion and provide guidance to these school Yogo teachers, in addition to checking the health of all pupils and students once a year. The Japanese school system also recognizes the important role that physicians play in promoting the optimal biopsychosocial well-being of children in the school setting. Regrettably, such check-ups are only for physical conditions, and not for mental health.

The school counsellor works closely with the school management in planning and implementing a school-wide counselling system. In contrast to Yogo teachers, Japanese school counsellors are employed part-time and, at the moment, are not assigned to every school (though the Ministry of Education sets a goal to allocate one school counsellor to every public school). Their responsibilities include: providing direct counselling intervention for students; conducting case consultations for school personnel and parents; training teachers and parents on counselling-related issues; and identifying, devising, and delivering specialized group guidance programmes for students who need additional help in the area of social and emotional development, as evidenced by social, emotional, and behavioural concerns presented by these students.

Creating a good network among the aforementioned unique school professionals—Yogo teachers, school counsellors, school physicians, and psychiatrists—who are focused on the care of young people, might be a very effective resource for achieving the early referral of students who require specialized care. The targets of early detection should not be limited to psychosis and related disorders, autism spectrum disorder (ASD), and attention deficit/hyperactivity disorder (ADHD); instead, all mental symptoms under clinical threshold such as Hikikomori [11] should be targeted. When considering how to improve youth mental health generally, we need to be attentive to the particular needs of young populations, especially during policy planning and service design.

'Il Bosco' integrated approach to youth mental health

A representative early intervention facility for young people in Japan is 'Il Bosco', where the authors work. This facility was founded in May 2007 at the Toho University Omori Medical Center in Tokyo. The unit is run according to an optimal treatment project (OTP) [1] that employs a multidisciplinary team and utilizes the cognitive remediation-orientated method advocated by Falloon et al.[12]. The service model includes early detection and intervention, repeated assessment, and psychoeducation. Treatment strategies consist of optimal pharmacotherapy based on four possible interventions (i.e. atypical neuroleptics, cognitive function training, cognitive behavioural therapy, and job coaching) as part of the final treatment programme. Cognitive function training is aimed at stimulating divergent thinking, mainly via paper- and computer-based tasks. It mainly targets deficits in divergent thinking, since interventions for divergent thinking have been previously found to improve negative symptoms and social functioning significantly in patients with schizophrenia [13]. Cognitive interventions to improve deficits in divergent thinking during the early stage of psychosis may maximize the chance for functional recovery; and such interventions may minimize the risk of future progression in a subset of people with ARMS, since divergent thinking is critical for generating solutions to various social problems and for navigating the complexities of social interactions.

The clients of 'Il Bosco' are restricted to ARMS or first-episode schizophrenia patients between the ages of 15 and 30 years. Almost ten years have passed since the opening of 'Il Bosco'. About 80 per cent of the patients have improved through participation in a rehabilitation programme that focuses on social cognition, and this has enabled them to return to their former workplaces or schools. We are currently developing some new programmes for cognitive rehabilitation and remediation, as well as a psychoeducation website for individuals with early psychosis.

References

1. **Organisation for Economic Co-operation and Development** (**OECD**). OECD reviews of health care quality: Japan—assessment and recommendations. OECD. 2014.
2. **Mizuno M**, **Murakami M.** Differences in strategies for implementing community-based psychiatry in Japan. In: **Lefley HP**, **Johnson DL**, editors. Family interventions in mental illness: international perspectives. Westport, CT: Praeger Publishers; 2002. p. 185–92.
3. **Mizuno M**, **Suzuki M**, **Matsumoto K**, **Murakami M**, **Takeshi K**, **Miyakoshi T**, et al. Clinical practice and research activities for early psychiatric intervention at Japanese leading centers. Early Interv Psychiatry. 2009; **3**:5–9.
4. **Mizuno M.** The duration of untreated schizophrenia and the epidemiological study on the prognosis. In: The Report for the Comprehensive Research on Disability Health and Welfare (H20-SEISHIN-IPPAN-010) from the Ministry of Health, Labour, and Welfare, Japan. 2011. p 7–35.
5. **Ministry of Health, Welfare, and Labour, Japan.** [Website for young adolescents providing information on early intervention]. 2016. Available from: http://www.mhlw.go.jp/kokoro/youth/
6. **Nishii H**, **Yamazawa R**, **Shimodera S**, **Suzuki M**, **Hasegawa T**, **Mizuno M.** Clinical and social determinants of a longer duration of untreated psychosis of schizophrenia in a Japanese population. Early Interv Psychiatry. 2010; **4**:182–8.
7. **Tsujino N**, **Katagiri N**, **Kobayashi H**, **Nemoto T**, **Mizuno M.** Recognition and decisions regarding the treatment of early psychosis by Japanese psychiatrists [in Japanese]. Seishin Igaku. 2010; **52**:1151–9.
8. **Kobayashi H**, **Nozaki A**, **Mizuno M.** Reliability of the structured interview for prodromal syndromes Japanese version (SIPS-J)[in Japanese]. Jpn Bull Soc Psychiatry. 2006; **15**:168–74.
9. **Kobayashi H**, **Nemoto T**, **Koshikawa H**, **Soon Y**, **Yamazawa R**, **Murakami M**, et al. A self-reported instrument for prodromal symptoms of psychosis: testing the clinical validity of the PRIME Screen-Revised (PS-R) in a Japanese population. Schizophr Res. 2008; **106**:356–62.
10. **Miyakoshi T**, **Matsumoto K**, **Ito F**, **Ohmuro N**, **Matsuoka H.** Application of the Comprehensive Assessment of At-Risk Mental States (CAARMS) to the Japanese

population: reliability and validity of the Japanese version of the CAARMS. Early Interv Psychiatry. 2009; **3**:123–30.

11. **Teo AR**. A new form of social withdrawal in Japan: a review of hikikomori. Int J Soc Psychiatry. 2010 Mar;**56**(2):178–85. doi: 10.1177/0020764008100629. Epub 2009 Jun 30.
12. **Falloon IRH, Montero I, Sungur M, Mastroeni A, Malm U, Economou M**, et al. Implementation of evidence-based treatment for schizophrenic disorders: two-year outcome of an international field trial of optimal treatment. World Psychiatry. 2004; **3**:104–9.
13. **Nemoto T, Yamazawa R, Kobayashi H, Fujita N, Chino B, Fujii C**, et al. Cognitive training for divergent thinking in schizophrenia: a pilot study. Prog Neuro-psychoph. 2009; **33**:1533–6.

Chapter 11

Family involvement in first-episode psychosis

The Indian scenario

Greeshma Mohan, R. Padmavati, and R. Thara

Introduction

The term 'family' is derived from the Latin word 'familia', denoting a household establishment, and refers to a 'group of individuals living together during important phases of their lifetime and bound to each other by biological and/or social and psychological relationship' [1]. India is a secular and pluralistic society characterized by tremendous cultural and ethnic diversity [2]. The family is the oldest and most important institution that has survived through the ages. Like most traditional, eastern societies, India is also a collectivist society that emphasizes family integrity, family loyalty, and family unity. More specifically, the character of collectivism is reflected in a greater readiness to cooperate with family members and extended kin on decisions affecting most aspects of life, including career choice, mate selection, marriage, and the upbringing of children. In collectivist or socio-centric societies, the individual gives way to the larger kinship and their identity is influenced by the kinship or the group they belong to. As in many other countries around the globe, rapid urbanization in India in the last two decades has brought about chaotic changes in social, economic, political, religious, and occupational spheres. There has been a progressive increase in nuclear families, more so in urban areas, with an associated progressive decrease in the number of household members [3].

It is well recognized that a majority of individuals with schizophrenia and related psychotic disorders live in the developing world, about seven to eight million in India alone [4]. The Determinants of Outcome of Severe Mental Disorder (DOSMeD) study found that acute psychosis is more prevalent in developing countries and among females [5]. The phenomenon of a better prognosis for schizophrenia in 'developing' than in 'developed' countries is 'the single most important finding of cultural differences in cross cultural research on mental health' [6]. The bulk of the evidence for this comes from three cross-national studies conducted by the World Health Organization (WHO) [5, 7–10]. Several criticisms have been levelled against this finding and a 2008 paper by Cohen et al. questioned the WHO studies by arguing that there is great variation in clinical outcomes even among 'developing' countries [11]. This resulted in a vibrant discussion on the topic of sociocultural factors and psychosis outcomes [12–16]. There have been calls for more carefully designed and better interpreted research studies. Several centres in India have studied prodrome or early psychosis in the past two decades [17–19]. Data from a first-episode psychoses project—started in 2007 at the Schizophrenia Research Foundation (SCARF), India, in collaboration with the Prevention and Early Intervention Programme for Psychoses (PEPP), Montreal, Canada—is currently being analysed.

It is well recognized that a first episode of psychosis typically occurs in late adolescence or young adulthood, and may well follow a prodromal period of approximately four years, which is characterized by the emergence of non-specific symptoms and functional decline. Further, an additional period of duration of untreated psychosis (DUP) is common; it is estimated to last an average of one to two years and is associated with worse outcome. The trajectory indicates that by the time a young person receives treatment for a first episode of psychosis, significant damage may have already occurred in almost all aspects of their lives. In this period, adverse behaviour and victimization are common. and pathways to care are indirect and tortuous [20]. Consequently, it is well known that psychotic illnesses cause immense suffering for patients and equally to their families and carers.

The role of the family therefore becomes apparent in India, with a population of more than one billion people and a paucity of trained personnel (the number of mental health professionals such as psychiatrists and psychologists not exceeding a total of 5,000 for the whole country). For such a huge population, the number of both clinical settings and service providers is grossly inadequate. Needless to say, a large part of mental healthcare therefore takes place in the community, making the family the primary care provider [3] and the source of support.

Also, with psychiatry putting the theory of the schizophrenogenic mother to rest [21], and with effective methods to handle expressed emotions being considered, the crucial and positive role that family plays in recovery is changing and emerging in a more unquestionable way [22]. Since families play such a highly significant role in the treatment of schizophrenia in India, family factors may hold the key to the question of why outcomes are better there, although these are yet to be substantiated.

The last decade or so has witnessed an upsurge of research on early intervention for psychotic disorders in India, as well as globally. Early intervention can minimize relapses and maximize recovery, as outcome in the early years significantly predicts the long-term illness course [23–25]. Research publications from India have described in greater depth the role of traditional Indian families and the efficacy of family interventions, but there is a definite paucity of research on the subject of 'family involvement'.

Review

In this chapter, we aim to provide a review of the findings emerging from several studies carried out on first-episode psychosis (FEP) patients at SCARF and other Indian centres.

SCARF—a non-profit, non-governmental organization in the south Indian city of Chennai—is also a WHO-collaborating centre for mental health research and training. The chapter refers to various studies carried out by SCARF over a period of some 30 years, many of which have been in collaboration with other international partners. SCARF has an outpatient department (OPD) manned by a multi-professional team. An average of 12 new patients and 100 review patients are seen in the OPD every day, and there are facilities to admit about 140 patients. A number of community outreach programmes also operate to detect first-episode patients, many of whom have remained untreated for long periods [26]. The other major centres which have published research in FEP include the National Institute of Mental Health and Neurological Sciences (NIMHANS), Bengaluru, and the All India Institute of Medical Sciences (AIIMS), New Delhi.

Keeping in mind that over 95 per cent of persons with psychotic disorders live with their families, we propose to outline the various ways in which families influence the course of FEP. The broad areas are:

1. Identification of prodromal symptoms and premorbid characteristics
2. Pathways to care/seeking help
3. Family needs
4. Family role in adherence and relapse prevention
5. Stigma and burden

Identifying prodromes and early signs and symptoms

Initiatives on early detection and early intervention, near-psychotic prodromal symptoms, as well as deficits of thought and perception, observable by the affected person himself, have been found to be particularly helpful in predicting the onset and progress of psychosis [27]. There is no doubt that if the individual with psychosis is living with the family, the family members are well placed to identify the prodromal phase of psychosis. Several studies (although not primarily addressing prodromes) have cited reports by families on very early changes in behaviours. In India, as already noted, inadequate mental health services, together with cultural factors, do not facilitate specialized prodrome services.

Research on FEP has reported on what families identified as 'different' behaviour traits. In SOFACOS [28]—a three-site study on first-episode schizophrenia funded by the Indian Council of Medical Research—family carers reported on childhood and adolescent behavioural traits such as extreme shyness, sensitivity, and difficulties in concentration, but they did not see these as precursors to developing a problem later in life. Over 60 per cent of families felt the patients had become well-adjusted by then.

A subsequent qualitative study through the narratives of relatives, explored early symptoms and identified two main clusters of behaviours as core symptoms: aggressiveness and withdrawal. Aggressiveness appeared to be emphasized by husbands, while withdrawal was particularly prominent in accounts by mothers [29]. Keshavan et al. reiterate this in a study on FEP in south India where the family members were interviewed extensively and only 7 per cent of the 300 had a discernible prodromal phase of psychosis [30]. They went on to ascribe this to the rather low levels of drug abuse in this sample along with a high level of tolerance for abnormal behaviours by families.

A more recent study from SCARF aimed to identify symptom clusters recognized by caregivers at illness onset in first-episode schizophrenia [17]. Caregivers, predominantly women, were assessed using a questionnaire adapted from the Psychiatric and Personal History Schedule. Principal component (PCP) analysis of the symptom data rated on the caregiver questionnaire indicated a four-factor solution—depressive, anxious, irritable, and vegetative factors. Caregivers (40 per cent) attributed present lifestyle as a possible causal factor to the onset of illness. These authors suggest that the caregiver's perception about mental illness and ability to identify early symptoms in clusters may have important treatment implications for developing and delivering early intervention programmes.

Pathways to care

As mentioned earlier, the well-recognized role of the family in the Indian scene is all-pervasive, influencing as it does the decision to seek help (when, where, and how), the nature of help (medical or non-medical depending upon explanatory models), the need to continue treatment, and other issues such as employment and marriage [4]. Recognition of prodromal or early psychotic symptoms and the attribution of cause by family members play a significant role in the access of mental healthcare services. Several studies on pathways to care have shown that access can include no access at all ('never treated'), religious healers, traditional medical systems, non-psychiatric medical services, or, much less frequently, psychiatric services [31–35].

An incidence and prevalence study of psychoses was carried out in a Chennai urban community [36]. This study reported that even the incident cases had a long DUP, with an average of over six years. This was despite the fact that patients were in the close vicinity of at least two state-run mental health facilities for which they did not have to pay anything. One of the interesting associations with longer DUP and delayed treatment was living in a joint family. The DUP was significantly lower in persons living in a nuclear family. The authors postulate that the presence of many members in the family, some being homemakers or retired persons, might result in better tolerance of abnormal behaviours [37] and perhaps lower expectations of the individual to contribute to the family income.

In the three-site study on first-episode schizophrenia mentioned earlier [28], only 21 per cent of 386 FEP patients in the three sites of Lucknow, Vellore, and Chennai had consulted a psychiatrist as the first contact for help. Over half (52 per cent) of the families in this sample had taken the patients to a religious or traditional healer as the first source of help. This can be explained by the explanatory models of illness held by the families and, to an extent, by the patients themselves. It is interesting to note, that while 66 per cent of family carers believed it could be some kind of mental disorder, many of them could not clearly elucidate what they thought might be the cause. Thirty per cent of the families had no explanation, while 20 per cent thought the family could be a causal factor for the illness. They also wondered if the upbringing of the child had something to do with the onset of the illness in the patient's early twenties, as he or she might seem quite normal before the onset. A few families referred to 'heredity', citing similar problems in other family members.

Data from an outpatient psychiatric clinic in northern India [31] showed that in the study group which had a mean 14-day time interval between onset of odd or threatening behaviours and accessing help, 70 per cent of them had first contacted traditional or religious healers and only 10 per cent first sought help from the psychiatric service. Campion and Bhugra [32] opined that the medical literature seldom mentions traditional healers despite their importance as the first line of treatment in developing countries.

Thirty years later, there does not seem to be much change in what families perceive to be the causes of psychotic disorders and those that determine the first port of help. Preliminary work in the INTREPID study, which looked at first-episode psychosis in a rural community, showed that all family carers of the 62 patients we interviewed sought the help of traditional and religious healers, thereby increasing the DUP [26]. Such observations thus emphasize the need to work with religious and faith healers in order to reduce the DUP.

Studies on pathways to care have underscored the importance of understanding the factors associated with them in order to develop strategies to improve detection and treatment of psychiatric disorders.

Needs of carers of first-episode psychosis patients

Parallel to understanding the family's role in recognizing early symptoms of a first episode of psychosis and seeking treatment, it is important to recognize that an understanding of the needs of the family is crucial in the process of treatment planning. In a study carried out at the National Institute of Mental Health and Neurological Sciences (NIMHANS) in the southern city of Bangalore, six prominent needs of carers of FEP patients were identified. Of these, the need for obtaining information on the illness and its management seemed to be the most important and easily satisfied of all. The socioeconomic class and educational qualifications of the carers seem to largely determine this need [19]. Next in importance, families expressed the need for follow-up services such as ongoing support/brief counselling and telephonic consultations. A few wanted the help of support groups, if available. They sought information on the various obtainable welfare measures and the processes for accessing them, on legal recourse in cases of disputes, and tips on management of the illness itself such as detecting early signs of relapse and side effects of medication.

The Madras Longitudinal Study was the follow-up of 90 patients recruited in the SOFACOS mentioned earlier. Since this was a follow-up of FEP patients, we decided to look at the changing patterns of care of these patients by the family members. This also reflected the changing needs of the carers. While the primary carers at intake were predominantly parents (82 per cent), not surprisingly, there was a shift as years rolled by and parents either died or became too old to care. The responsibility then shifted to spouses, the children of those who were married, and to siblings and other members of the extended family. The siblings' primary role was noted as providing financial support or in being assertive towards the patients when they are uncooperative. The parents themselves expressed concern that siblings who had their own families to care for may not be able to provide quality care to the ill sibling. The initial focus was on management of symptoms, relapse, and ensuring adherence, while later on, it was looking after the physical health needs, financial needs, and security (more so, in the case of women) (Mohan et al. in preparation).

Relapse and recovery: the role of the family

A low expressed emotion in families of schizophrenia patients making the first contact with a treatment facility was demonstrated at Chandigarh [38]. In a subsequent report, Leff et al. (1990) followed up 86 per cent of the Chandigarh group of patients at the end of two years [39]. In contrast to the one-year findings, the global EE index at initial interview did not predict relapse of schizophrenia over the next two years. However, there was a significant association between initial hostility and subsequent relapse. Although the concept of expressed emotions did not attract attention for subsequent research [40], the family in India continues to anchor the interventions in psychosis. Literature on recovery from serious mental illnesses has universally identified several factors—such as the environment which enables personal growth, resilience to stress, and being believed in, listened to, and understood by families, friends, and health and social service personnel—that are very helpful to people on the road to recovery [41].

The role of family members in interventions, as well as in maintaining recovery, is widely acknowledged. Unpublished data from a focus-group discussion (FGD) conducted in 2009 at SCARF with eight young patients with FEP revealed interesting aspects of family involvement. All but one of these young patients were students, and the one who was not, was employed. Families were seen to play key roles in the early stages of the illness when help is first being sought and in providing long-term support to maintain recovery. The narratives reflected several different important and specific roles played by family members but predominantly in relation to adherence to medication, watching out for relapse, or in overall functioning:

> As patients, we will not be able to remember and take medicines regularly . . . family members will remind us to take medicines. (Patient 5)
>
> While on treatment, parents monitor us, and they can identify the changes (in behaviour) before and after. In my family . . . they keep observing me. (Patient 2)
>
> My family cares for me. They won't get irritated with me . . . won't wonder why he is doing this. They understand that it is due to mental illness that I behave oddly at times . . . and they won't feel worried about it. (Patient1)

All patients endorsed the role of family members in supporting them in their work and studies:

> If I say I want to take rest and won't go for work, my family will understand and co-operate. They won't compel me to join work immediately. So, I am not stressed. (Patient 5)
>
> I am not able to study since I have a problem in concentration. I told my mother I will study next year, she said okay. She didn't force me to go to college. She understood my problem and supported me. (Patient 7)

Stigma and confidentiality

While issues pertaining to confidentiality and stigma appear to be challenging throughout the course of a mental illness, it is particularly perplexing in young people with psychosis. Much of the literature on stigma deals with chronic mental illnesses and has not been robustly addressed in FEP.

In an unpublished study on stigma carried out at SCARF, one emerging theme was the reluctance to disclose. One mother of a young college-going daughter had this to say:

> I don't want the college to know about S taking treatment here … I am afraid that the college will ask her to discontinue … it is important that my daughter completes her education and starts work … She has to support the family … And, later other family members get to know—then I will have difficulty getting her married!

A number of similar concerns are expressed by families accessing routine clinical services for the FEP group. This is more obvious with young women who are single, since the families are keen to get them married as soon as they see signs of recovery. One such example is of a young girl, aged 18, who was treated for the first episode at SCARF and recovered within three months of starting her on treatment. The family decided to discontinue treatment and quickly got her married. Two months later, she was brought back to the facility, pregnant and floridly symptomatic. The family's key request was that the team should make no contact with the spouse, since the girl's marriage would be at stake. Such situations pose a great ethical challenge for the treating team.

Discussion

The incidence, impact, and consequences of mental health problems are well known. What is less known and appreciated is the tremendous but often invisible role that family members have to and can play. However, in the research field, there appears to be a positive change in the way the role of families is perceived, from the days of the schizophrenogenic mother and double-bind to recognizing their role as not only the major carers of patients with mental illnesses but also as co-producers, working with clinicians and mental health professionals. This has also led to research measuring the burden of caregiving. Our work in following up FEP patients over several decades shows there is not much change in the family's role as years roll by.

In India, family members who care for relatives with mental health problems serve a variety of crucial roles and, through their involvement in treatment, they may act as informal case managers, provide crisis intervention, and enhance adherence to treatment choices, leading to decreased rates of hospitalization and relapse and increased rates of recovery. When compared to countries in the West, support from the Indian government for mental illness is very minimal and families provide financial support, housing, and assistance with activities of daily living [42]. This has direct implications in determining the needs of the families and delivering these. Many families would like information on the illness and its management [19]. Often, in busy outpatient departments with large clinical loads, little information—other than urging them to ensure treatment adherence—is provided to families. Non-governmental organizations can play a major role in this task. To ensure that the families remain involved and engaged, looking after a patient following their psychotic episode and for years to follow, we need to work with the families and provide them with the information and support they require.

The finding that the DUP in incident cases was less in persons from nuclear families, rather than joint and extended families, is indeed intriguing. It makes one wonder about the commonly held belief here that living in joint families provides a lot of support and care. At the same time, does it also delay help-seeking due to the shared tolerance and varying views of the different family members [37]? As mentioned earlier, it may be that in a nuclear family, individual patients are expected to earn an income and their inability to do so may bring them to attention and help-seeking quicker.

There are, of course, issues to do with privacy and confidentiality. Often, in clinical settings in India, the patient will be brought to the clinic accompanied by several individuals, thereby raising challenges related to confidentiality regarding their condition and therapeutic interventions. Stigma associated with mental disorders also plays a role, irrespective of the duration of illness. Emerging research on stigma in FEP reflects on self-stigma [43, 44], and affiliated stigma in caregivers can manifest as increased stress and emotional distress [44, 45].

These insights have clear implications for addressing the pertinent issue of involving family members as partners in treatment and recovery. Stigma research reiterates the role of psycho-education and other interventions to cope with the stigma for families of persons in a FEP.

Conclusion

There is no doubt that, as summarized by Chadda and Deb [2], in a situation where mental health resources are scarce, families form a valuable support system, which can be extremely helpful in managing stressful situations. Yet, this resource is not adequately and appropriately utilized. Clinicians in India do routinely take time to educate family members of a patient about the illness and the importance of medication, but apart from this information exchange, the utilization of the family in treatment is minimal. Therefore, recognizing families as partners in care, rehabilitation, and recovery is the primary need. Findings from FEP research in developing countries have important clinical and systemic implications. They throw light on the role of the family in the recovery process in FEP, and qualitative data can be used to develop a quantitative tool which will tap into the levels of family involvement and other dynamics. The ultimate goal will be to help provide a service which is sensitive, appropriate, and accessible to the needs of the patients and family members who are dealing with an episode of psychotic illness for the first time.

References

1. **Sethi BB.** Family as a potent therapeutic force. Indian J Psychiatry. 1989; **31**(1):22.
2. **Chadda RK, Deb KS.** Indian family systems, collectivistic society and psychotherapy. Indian J Psychiatry. 2013; **55**(Suppl 2):S299.
3. **Avasthi A.** Preserve and strengthen family to promote mental health. Indian J Psychiatry. 2010; **52**(2):113.
4. **Thara R, Padmavati R, Srinivasan TN.** Focus on psychiatry in India. Br J Psychiatry J Ment Sci. 2004 Apr; 184:366–73.
5. **Jablensky A, Sartorius N, Ernberg G, Anker M, Korten A, Cooper JE**, et al. Schizophrenia: manifestations, incidence and course in different cultures. A World Health Organization ten-country study. Psychol Med Monogr Suppl. 1992; **20**:1–97. Available from: https://www.cambridge.org/core/journals/psychological-medicine-monograph-supplement/article/schizophrenia-manifestations-incidence-and-course-in-different-cultures-a-world-health-organization-ten-country-study/4C45DDB6CAB367EB9A2DD91E4FEF13C9
6. **Lin K-M, Kleinman AM.** Psychopathology and clinical course of schizophrenia: a cross-cultural perspective. Schizophr Bull. 1988; **14**(4):555–67.
7. **Hopper K, Wanderling J.** Revisiting the developed versus developing country distinction in course and outcome in schizophrenia: results from ISoS, the WHO collaborative follow-up project. Schizophr Bull. 2000; **26**(4):835–46.
8. **Harrison G, Hopper KIM, Craig T, Laska E, Siegel C, Wanderling J**, et al. Recovery from psychotic illness: a 15- and 25-year international follow-up study. Br J Psychiatry. 2001; **178**(6):506–17.

9. **Leff J, Sartorius N, Jablensky A, Korten A, Ernberg G.** The International Pilot Study of Schizophrenia: five-year follow-up findings. Psychol Med. 1992; **22**(01):131–45. Available from: http://journals.cambridge.org/article_S0033291700032797
10. **Sartorius N, Gulbinat W, Harrison G, Laska E, Siegel C.** Long-term follow-up of schizophrenia in 16 countries. Soc Psychiatry Psychiatr Epidemiol. 1996; **31**(5):249–58. Available from: http://www.springerlink.com/index/R74850292W037L45.pdf
11. **Cohen A, Patel V, Thara R, Gureje O.** Questioning an axiom: better prognosis for schizophrenia in the developing world? Schizophr Bull. 2008; **34**(2):229–44. Available from: http://schizophreniabulletin.oxfordjournals.org/content/34/2/229.short
12. **Kleinman A.** Commentary on Alex Cohen et al: 'Questioning an axiom: better prognosis for schizophrenia in the developing world'. Schizophr Bull. 2007; **34**(2):249–50.
13. **Jablensky A, Sartorius N.** What did the WHO studies really find? Schizophr Bull. 2008; **34**(2):253–5. Available from: https://academic.oup.com/schizophreniabulletin/article-abstract/34/2/253/1925460
14. **Leff J.** Comment on paper by Cohen, Patel, Thara, and Gureje. Schizophr Bull. 2008; **34**(2):251–2.
15. **Bromet EJ.** Cross-national comparisons: problems in interpretation when studies are based on prevalent cases. Schizophr Bull. 2008; **34**(2):256–7. Available from: https://academic.oup.com/schizophreniabulletin/article-abstract/34/2/256/1925657
16. **McGrath J.** Dissecting the heterogeneity of schizophrenia outcomes. Schizophr Bull. 2007; **34**(2):247–8. Available from: https://academic.oup.com/schizophreniabulletin/article-abstract/34/2/247/1924806
17. **Tharoor H, Ganesh A.** Symptoms at onset in first episode schizophrenia: caregivers perspectives. Indian J Psychol Med. 2015 Dec; **37**(4):399–402.
18. **Rangaswamy T, Mangala R, Mohan G, Joseph J, John S.** Intervention for first episode psychosis in India—the SCARF experience. Asian J Psychiatry. 2012 Mar; **5**(1):58–62.
19. **Udgiri SM, Nirmala BP, Thirthalli J.** The care-giving needs of carers of persons with first episode of psychosis: exploratory qualitative findings from India. J Psychosoc Rehabil Ment Health. 2017; **4**(2):159–70.
20. **Corcoran C, Gerson R, Sills-Shahar R, Nickou C, McGlashan T, Malaspina D**, et al. Trajectory to a first episode of psychosis: a qualitative research study with families. Early Interv Psychiatry. 2007; **1**(4):308–15. Available from: http://onlinelibrary.wiley.com/doi/10.1111/j.1751-7893.2007.00041.x/full
21. **Neill J.** Whatever became of the schizophrenogenic mother? Am J Psychother. 1990; **44**(4):499–505.
22. **Amaresha AC**, Venkatasubramanian G. Expressed emotion in schizophrenia: an overview. Indian J Psychol Med. 2012; **34**(1):12. Available from: https://www.ncbi.nlm.nih.gov/pmc/articles/PMC3361836/
23. **Birchwood M, Todd P, Jackson C.** Early intervention in psychosis: the critical-period hypothesis. Int Clin Psychopharmacol. 1998; **13**:S31–S40. Available from: http://journals.lww.com/intclinpsychopharm/Abstract/1998/01001/Early_intervention_in_psychosis__the.6.aspx
24. **Malla AK, Norman RM, Manchanda R, Ahmed MR, Scholten D, Harricharan R**, et al. One year outcome in first episode psychosis: influence of DUP and other predictors.

Schizophr Res. 2002; **54**(3):231–42. Available from: http://www.sciencedirect.com/science/article/pii/S0920996401002547

25. **Penn DL, Waldheter EJ, Perkins DO, Mueser KT, Lieberman JA.** Psychosocial treatment for first-episode psychosis: a research update. Am J Psychiatry. 2005; **62**(12):2220. Available from: http://ajp.psychiatryonline.org/doi/abs/10.1176/appi.ajp.162.12.2220
26. **Morgan C, John S, Esan O, Hibben M, Patel V, Weiss H,** et al. The incidence of psychoses in diverse settings, INTREPID (2): a feasibility study in India, Nigeria, and Trinidad. Psychol Med. 2016 Jul; **46**(9):1923–33.
27. **Hambrecht M.** Emerging psychosis and the family. ISRN Psychiatry. 2012; 2012:219642.
28. **Verghese A, Dube KC, John JK, Kumar N, Nandi DN, Parhee R,** et al. Factors associated with the course and outcome of schizophrenia a multicentred follow-up study: result of five year follow-up. Indian J Psychiatry. 1990 Jul; **32**(3):211–6.
29. **Corin E, Thara R, Padmavati R.** Shadows of culture in psychosis in south India: a methodological exploration and illustration. Int Rev Psychiatry. 2005; **17**(2):75–81.
30. **Keshavan MS, Shrivastava A, Gangadhar BN.** Early intervention in psychotic disorders: challenges and relevance in the Indian context. Indian J Psychiatry. 2010 Jan; **52**(Suppl 1):S153–8.
31. **Sagar R, Pattanayak RD, Chandrasekaran R, Chaudhury PK, Deswal BS, Singh RL,** et al. Twelve-month prevalence and treatment gap for common mental disorders: findings from a large-scale epidemiological survey in India. Indian J Psychiatry. 2017; **59**(1):46.
32. **Campion J, Bhugra D.** Experiences of religious healing in psychiatric patients in south India. Soc Psychiatry Psychiatr Epidemiol. 1997 May; **32**(4):215–21.
33. **Cohen A, Padmavati R, Hibben M, Oyewusi S, John S, Esan O,** et al. Concepts of madness in diverse settings: a qualitative study from the INTREPID project. BMC Psychiatry. 2016 Nov 9; **16**(1):388.
34. **Padmavathi R, Rajkumar S, Srinivasan TN.** Schizophrenic patients who were never treated—a study in an Indian urban community. Psychol Med. 1998 Sep; **28**(5):1113–17.
35. **Phang CK, Marhani M, Salina AA.** Help-seeking pathways for in-patients with first-episode psychosis in Hospital Kuala Lumpur. Malays J Med Health Sci. 2011; 7(2):37–44.
36. **Rajkumar S, Padmavathi R, Thara R, Menon MS.** Incidence of schizophrenia in an urban community in madras. Indian J Psychiatry. 1993 Jan; **35**(1):18–21.
37. **Srinivasan Tirupati N, Rangaswamy T, Raman P.** Duration of untreated psychosis and treatment outcome in schizophrenia patients untreated for many years. Aust N Z J Psychiatry. 2004; **38**(5):339–43. Available from: http://journals.sagepub.com/doi/abs/10.1080/j.1440-1614.2004.01361.x
38. **Wig NN, Menon DK, Bedi H, Leff J, Kuipers L, Ghosh A,** et al. Expressed emotion and schizophrenia in north India. II. Distribution of expressed emotion components among relatives of schizophrenic patients in Aarhus and Chandigarh. Br J Psychiatry. 1987 Aug; **151**:160–5.

39. **Leff J, Wig NN, Bedi H, Menon DK, Kuipers L, Korten A**, et al. Relatives' expressed emotion and the course of schizophrenia in Chandigarh. A two-year follow-up of a first-contact sample. Br J Psychiatry. 1990 Mar; **156**:351–6.
40. **Murthy RS.** Family interventions and empowerment as an approach to enhance mental health resources in developing countries. World Psychiatry. 2003 Feb; **2**(1):35–7.
41. **Jacob KS.** Recovery model of mental illness: a complementary approach to psychiatric care. Indian J Psychol Med. 2015; **37**(2):117.
42. **Kallivayalil RA, Sudhakar S.** Effectiveness of a new low-cost psychosocial rehabilitative model to reduce burden of disease among persons with severe mental illness: an interventional follow-up study. Indian J Psychiatry. 2018; **60**(1):65.
43. **McCann TV, Lubman DI, Clark E.** Responding to stigma: first-time caregivers of young people with first-episode psychosis. Psychiatr Serv. 2011; **62**(5):548–50.
44. **Chen ES, Chang WC, Hui CL, Chan SK, Lee EHM, Chen EY.** Self-stigma and affiliate stigma in first-episode psychosis patients and their caregivers. Soc Psychiatry Psychiatr Epidemiol. 2016; **51**(9):1225–31.
45. **Sadath A, Muralidhar D, Varambally S, Jose JP, Gangadhar BN.** Caregiving and help seeking in first episode psychosis: a qualitative study. J Psychosoc Rehabil Ment Health. 2014; **1**(2):47–53.

Chapter 12

From principles to practice

Translating the philosophy of early intervention to individuals with emerging bipolar disorders

Jan Scott

Introduction

Bipolar disorders (BD) are severe, persistent mental disorders characterized by recurrent episodes of mania, hypomania, and depression, separated by inter-episode periods of euthymia or residual symptoms. Globally, the lifetime prevalence of BD is estimated at about 2.5 per cent of the world's population, and the peak age at onset (AAO) of BD is late adolescence and early adulthood [1, 2]. In individuals under 25 years old, BD is ranked as the fourth most burdensome health condition worldwide [3]. The early AAO, persistence, and socioeconomic burden of BD emphasize why it is important to determine how to identify and intervene early in these disorders [4].

In the *DSM-5*, BD and related disorders are deliberately placed between psychotic and depressive disorders, in recognition of their place as a bridge between these diagnoses in terms of shared phenomenology, family history, and genetic liability [5]. Bipolar I disorder (BD-I) corresponds to the classic descriptions of manic-depressive illness (episodes of mania and depression, with or without psychotic features), and this diagnosis is one of the most reliable in psychiatry. However, the diagnosis of BD-II (hypomania and depression) and other manifestations (BD spectrum) show relatively poor inter-rater agreement.

Whilst the diagnostic criteria for BD are applicable for adolescents and adults, in some countries these criteria are applied to children [5]. Debate about the validity of diagnosing mania in children spans more than half a century (e.g. [6]), and the rapid increase in rates of paediatric BD in the USA is not reflected in community, epidemiological, or clinical studies internationally [7–9].

As such, this chapter will focus on the peak AAO of adult-pattern BD (onsets between 15 and 25 years).

Among individuals diagnosed with BD there are a wide variety of clinical presentations; also, patients may or may not have a family history of mood disorders, a personal biography complicated by traumatic life events, or co-morbid mental disorders [5]. In practice, this means that patients given a diagnosis of BD on cross-sectional assessment may show considerable individual differences in longitudinal outcomes and/or the stability of the diagnosis [4]. In an era of early intervention and personalized treatment, it is important to acknowledge the lack of predictive validity of most international diagnostic systems and their failure to truly guide treatment approaches [10]. As such, many researchers suggest that it is useful to augment traditional diagnostic approaches with models such as clinical staging, which are used routinely in general medicine (e.g. [11–16]). This is especially true when working with youth who often present with less stable, less well-defined syndromes [17].

Clinical staging models usually identify where an individual exists on a continuum from an asymptomatic 'at-risk' state (stage 0), to 'early illness' (stages 1 and 2), through to 'end-stage' disease (stages 3 and 4). In general medicine, treatment selection differs with stage of illness and is initiated before an individual develops a full syndromal disorder (which usually equates to stage 2). Thus, staging can be viewed as a more refined concept than cross-sectional diagnosis [15], and it actively promotes greater attention to indicated prevention strategies (e.g. interventions for individuals at ultra-high risk (UHR) of developing psychosis or BD) and has shaped the underlying principles of early intervention in psychosis (EIP) services [11, 14, 18]. McGorry and colleagues [19] suggest that the main goals of EIP can be operationalized as:

1. Reducing the delay to initiation of treatment by:
   i. Reducing the duration of untreated illness (DUI) or duration of untreated psychosis (DUP).
   ii. Detecting individuals at UHR of developing psychosis.
2. Providing optimal and specific management for the early phase of the illness by:
   i. Offering age- and stage-appropriate interventions.
   ii. Continuing input during a 'critical period' (about 2–5 years post onset).

This chapter now explores the key elements of EIP from the perspective of BD.

Current understanding of the duration of untreated bipolar

The concepts of DUP (time from first psychotic symptom to initiation of adequate antipsychotic treatment) and DUI (late prodrome until treatment) represent potentially modifiable factors and, as such, have played a critical part in the introduction of EIP and proactive approaches to case identification [20]. Meta-analyses have demonstrated that the mean DUP is between 67–124 weeks; however, most research has focused on schizophrenia, while affective disorders have been largely excluded from studies (e.g. [21]).

A meta-analysis by Scott [20] of nearly 30 studies (n=>9000) concluded that the median DUB was about six years. However, whilst this estimate had face validity, she suggested caution was needed because BD studies were usually smaller than those included in schizophrenia research, the DUI and DUB were operationalized in different ways, and there were differences in definitions of 'appropriate treatment' for BD, diagnostic assessments, and representativeness of the sample (e.g. self-identified cases, clinical samples, range of BD subtypes included), and so on.

Despite methodological heterogeneity, detailed studies of the DUB in large, well-characterized, clinically representative samples have demonstrated a similar set of key 'milestones' in the pathway from initial onset of symptoms up until treatment for BD. As shown in Fig. 12.1, Drancourt and colleagues [22] estimated that the mean DUI was just less than ten years (median six years). There was a gap of about three years between the first mood episode (often a depressive episode) and the first psychotropic treatment. During the next two to three years, most individuals were in contact with health services because of a first suicide attempt or because of psychiatric hospitalization. Despite these clinical contacts, a further three to five years elapsed before individuals were prescribed a recognized mood stabilizer—findings which reflect those of other studies. Delineating DUB milestones exposes the problems that exist in current clinical pathways, but also suggests that the DUB can be reduced by modifications of attitudes, skills, and/or knowledge of help-seeking youth and health professionals.

Identifying individuals at risk of bipolar disorders or with emerging bipolar disorders

In older adults, self-report instruments, such as the MDQ (Mood Disorders Questionnaire) and the HCL (Hypomania Checklist), have been used to detect signs and symptoms of BD in undiagnosed cases. Whilst these tools have

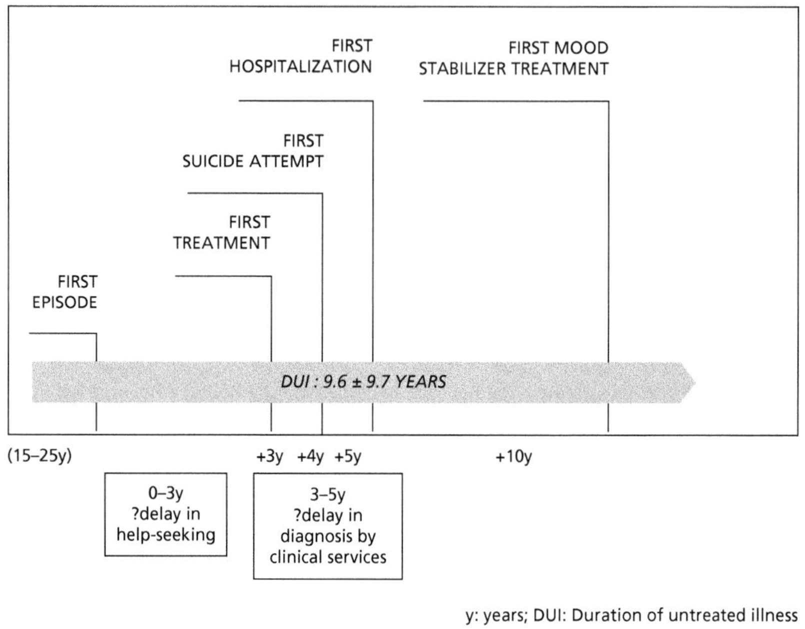

Fig. 12.1 Schematic representation of key milestones in the time period when bipolar disorder is untreated.

Adapted from *Acta Psychiatrica Scandinavica*, 127, 2, Drancourt N, Etain B, Lajnef M, Henry C, Raust A, Cochet B, et al., Duration of untreated bipolar disorder: missed opportunities on the long road to optimal treatment, pp. 136–144. Copyright (2013) John Wiley and Sons.

modest specificity in adults [23], they perform poorly as screening tools for identifying youth at risk of or with subthreshold BD symptoms [24].

At the other end of the age spectrum, very early detection of children at long-term risk of BD is hampered by the lack of specificity of the initial presentations in those who eventually develop BD and the lack of transdiagnostic data to allow better characterization of any BD-specific phenotypes [5, 25]. Also, it is not straightforward to differentiate normal temperament and transient behavioural changes in young adults from psychopathology indicative of an emerging severe mental disorder (e.g. [26]). Of course, many cohort studies do not examine family history of BD; studies of offspring of parents with BD (OSBD) demonstrate that they have a greater risk of developing BD than offspring of healthy controls and that the AAO of any mood disorder is often earlier in BD offspring (e.g. [27]). However, family history of BD alone is less helpful in differentiating early manifestations of a future (BD) illness trajectory when OSBD are compared to 'positive' controls such as the offspring of parents with schizophrenia (e.g. [28]).

The reliable and valid identification of a specific 'bipolar prodrome' is difficult because of the non-specific nature of early psychiatric symptoms (including transient (hypo)manic symptoms in adolescents), and the difficulty in predicting whether early onset depression will evolve into a unipolar disorder (UP) or BD (e.g. [29–31]). However, as shown in Fig. 12.2, recent progress has been made in identifying bipolar at-risk (BAR) criteria that incorporate a similar combination of a limited set of state, trait, and familial characteristics as used in UHR criteria for psychosis [32]. The risk of transition from BAR to BD is about 20–25 per cent over 12–18 months (compared to 1 per cent in those who do not meet BAR criteria), which is comparable to the risk of transition from UHR to first-episode psychosis over 24 months.

Bechdolf et al.'s [32, 33] BAR assessment tool has good reliability and incorporates generic risk factors (e.g. being in the peak AAO range for BD onset) alongside a set of specific criteria: namely, cyclothymia co-occurring with depression, subthreshold mania, and depression co-occurring with genetic risk (i.e. family history of BD). Scott and colleagues [25] explored the clinical utility and discriminant validity of the BAR criteria for predicting early transition to BD (ET-BD) in youth with early onset depression. The BAR criteria were extended to include five additional factors that have been shown to potentially discriminate between UP and ET-BD: namely, psychomotor retardation, evidence of psychotic symptoms during one or more mood episodes, atypical

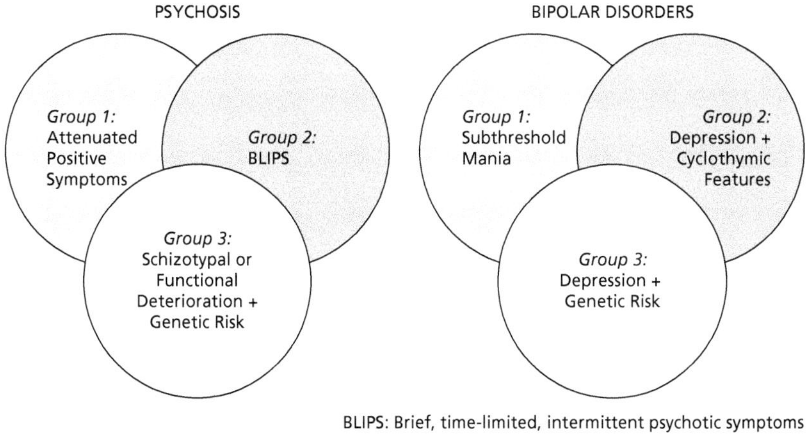

Fig. 12.2 Schematic representation of ultra-high risk (UHR) criteria for psychosis and bipolar at-risk (BAR) criteria in help-seeking young adults.

Adapted from *Journal of Affective Disorders*, 127, Bechdolf A, Nelson B, Cotton SM, Chanen A, Thompson A, Kettle J, et al., A preliminary evaluation of the validity of at-risk criteria for bipolar disorders in help-seeking adolescents and young adults, pp. 316–320. Copyright (2010) with permission from Elsevier.

depression features, family history of mood disorders in multiple generations, and family history of other mood and alcohol and substance use disorders.

Scott et al. [25] also examined the performance of the extended BAR criteria using the Clinical Utility Index (CUI), which assesses the discriminatory ability of a factor or criterion in the context of its overall rate of occurrence in the study population [34]. Basically, the CUI+ represents an estimate of the utility of a symptom or risk factor in case-finding, whilst the CUI– reflects the utility for screening out non-cases. As shown in Table 12.1, the original BAR criteria and two of the five additional risk factors significantly discriminated between ET-BD cases and UP controls. The key items (in order of magnitude of odds ratios) were subthreshold mania, cyclothymia, atypical depression, family history of BD, and evidence of probable antidepressant-emergent elation. However, the CUI scores suggest that cyclothymia had clinical utility for both case-finding and screening, whilst other items had better utility for screening only. For instance, subthreshold mania has a moderate CUI+ grading and a good CUI– grading, whilst probable antidepressant-emergent elation demonstrated a fair CUI+ but a good CUI– grading.

Table 12.1 Prevalence and performance (clinical utility and number needed to screen; NNS) of selected putative risk factors for bipolarity in differentiating between cases with early transition to bipolar disorders and controls with unipolar disorders

	ET-BD (N=50)	**UP (N=50)**	**Odds ratio (95% CI)**	**Clinical rule-in accuracy (CUI+)**	**Clinical rule-out accuracy (CUI–)**	**Overall clinical utility**
Cyclothymia	39	10	14.2 (5.4, 37.2)	Good	Good	Case-finding & screening
Subthreshold mania	26	3	16.9 (4.7, 61.8)	Moderate	Good	Screening
Family history of BD	12	2	7.6 (1.6, 35.9)	Poor	Good	Screening
Probable antidepressant-emergent elation	21	8	3.4 (1.2, 4.9)	Fair	Good	Screening
Atypical depression	25	4	11.5 (3.6, 36.7)	Fair	Good	Screening

ET-BD: Early transition to bipolar disorder; UP: unipolar disorder; 95% CI = 95% confidence intervals; CUI = Clinical Utility Index.

Adapted from *Schizophrenia*. Bulletin, 43, 4, Scott J, Marwaha S, Ratheesh A, Macmillan I, Yung AR, Morriss R, et al., Bipolar At-risk Criteria: An Examination of Which Clinical Features Have Optimal Utility for Identifying Youth at Risk of Early Transition From Depression to Bipolar Disorders, pp. 737–744. © The Author 2016. Published by Oxford University Press on behalf of the Maryland Psychiatric Research Center.

High-benefit, low-risk interventions for use during the critical period

The previous sections of this chapter suggest that significant progress is being made in our understanding of the DUB, BAR criteria, and predictive validity of other risk syndromes for future BD. The other important EIP principle described is the development of interventions that are appropriate for the critical period. Evidence demonstrates that early intervention strategies are more developed in depression and psychosis than in BD, and several EIP studies have extended interventions beyond the first illness episode towards the 'ultra-high risk' stages of illness [4].

In BD, interviews with asymptomatic OSBD and with adults with established disease suggest differences in opinions about when to commence interventions with individuals at above-average risk of developing BD, and a lack of consensus on what models of intervention might be offered [35]. Notably, parents with BD were keen on the provision of specialist services for offspring, even if their children were asymptomatic. In contrast, the offspring themselves expressed ambivalence about provision of dedicated services (reporting a preference for non-clinical peer support or generic inputs, which they regarded as less stigmatizing), and did not want interventions unless they experienced problems. Davidson and Scott note that the findings, whilst not definitive, reinforce the need to engage young people in the dialogue about service developments and not to rely on the opinions of significant others or older adult advocates.

Regarding low-risk, high-benefit interventions for the critical period in BD, it is conceivable that new medications could fit into this treatment specification. To date, there are no studies of specific pharmacotherapy for BAR or emerging BD. Further, it is not appropriate to simply prescribe medications that are used for adults with established illness to these youth [12, 16]. This is partly because there is no evidence that the medications used for late-stage BD will be helpful to individuals with subsyndromal BD, but also because it is ethically questionable to prescribe these medications to individuals fulfilling BAR criteria when, at most, only 20–30 per cent will develop syndromal BD [33]. In contrast to the paucity of new drug developments, there are several reviews that examine the benefits of psychological treatments for emerging BD. For instance, Vallarino et al. [36] recently undertook an 'evidence mapping' exercise to identify ongoing and completed studies that targeted psychological interventions at youth with recent-onset and first-episode BD, as well as individuals at risk of developing BD (such as symptomatic offspring of parents with BD, or youth who fulfil other BAR criteria). Interventions for the latter were especially

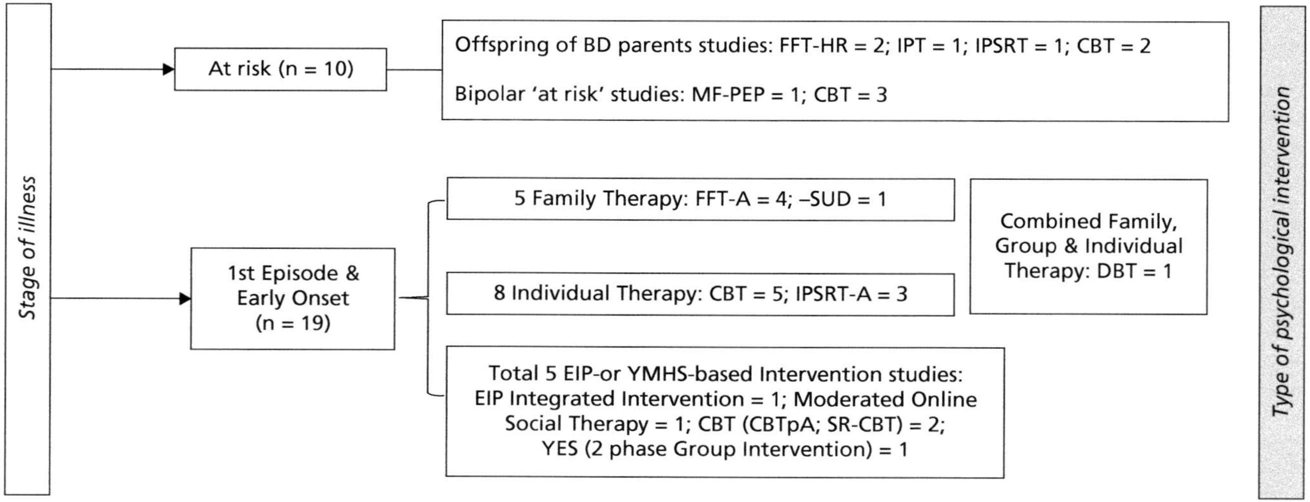

Fig. 12.3 Evidence map of 29 studies of psychological therapies for early stages of bipolar disorders.

BD: bipolar disorders; CBT: cognitive behaviour therapy; CBT-pA : psychosis, adolescents; SR-CBT: social recovery; DBT: dialectical behaviour therapy; EIP: early intervention in psychosis; IPT: interpersonal therapy; IPRST: interpersonal social rhythms therapy; IPSRT-A: adolescents; FFT: family-focused treatment; FFT-HR: high risk; FFT-A: adolescents; FFT-SUD: substance use disorder; MF-PEP: multi-family psychoeducation psychotherapy; YES: youth early intervention study; YMHS: youth mental health service.

Adapted from *Lancet Psychiatry*, 2, 6, Vallarino M, Henry C, Etain B, Gehue L, Macneil C, Scott E, et al., An evidence map of psychosocial interventions for the earliest stages of bipolar disorder, pp. 548–63.

sought out as, traditionally, these individuals have been excluded from mental health services [16].

As shown in Fig. 12.3, Vallarino et al. [36] identified 29 completed or ongoing studies, ranging from small case series to larger, multi-centre randomized controlled clinical trials. Ten studies focused on BAR or offspring of parents with BD, and five others targeted individuals experiencing their first episode of BD. Most of the established therapies for BD—such as family-focused treatment (FFT), interpersonal social rhythm therapy (IPSRT), and cognitive behaviour therapy (CBT)—had been used, although it was noticeable that no study has yet used a classic group psychoeducation programme. Vallarino et al. [36] noted that the translation of models of therapy that are widely used with older adults with established BD, to youth with emerging BD, had mostly focused on age-appropriate modifications, with limited attempts to introduce 'stage-appropriate' interventions (i.e. therapy techniques that specifically address risk factors for transition from subsyndromal to full syndromal disorders) or to consider how to tackle co-occurring problems, such as alcohol and substance misuse.

Overall, there was evidence of the positive effects of therapy on acute symptoms, such as anxiety or depression, on self-esteem and self-concept, and on social functioning. However, sample sizes and limited duration of study follow-ups meant that conclusions could not be reached on therapy effects on manic symptoms or transition rates. Interestingly, there was no evidence that BD-specific therapies (e.g. IPSRT, FFT) were more effective than transdiagnostic psychological interventions (such as social skills training or activity groups) offered to heterogeneous cases presenting to EIP or youth mental health services. Whilst this may indicate that 'generic' approaches can be recommended for individuals with emerging BD during the critical period, it is important to bear in mind that this field is under-researched and the picture may change in future [37].

Conclusions

A search of established databases (such as PubMed) over the last decade identified over 1,800 papers on clinical staging models of psychosis and EIP services, but less than 800 papers on the same topics in BD. This reflects how research in BD lags behind that in psychosis and partly explains why the understanding of and health service initiatives for early intervention in BD are in their infancy [4, 20]. In some ways, this is disappointing, as individuals with emerging BD constitute the second largest group of patients attending EIP, and BD is equally, if not more, burdensome to society than schizophrenia and possibly even more preventable [38]. More encouraging is the fact that it is now acknowledged that the degree of disability experienced by youth with recent-onset mood disorders has been underestimated [18], and a consensus is emerging on the rationale for intervening early in BD.

Studies are examining key milestones in the 'DUB pathway' and suggesting strategies that can be implemented to encourage help-seeking, to develop and employ appropriate BAR screening tools, and to increase early access to specialist assessment of youth with recurrent, early-onset depressive episodes who may be at increased risk of BD [4, 25, 32]. The latter is relevant, as it is a significant challenge to accurately categorize early, subtle presentations of BD within the current diagnostic frameworks and to exclude other conditions such as borderline personality disorder and substance use disorders [4].

Given the high prevalence of depression, but relatively low incidence rate of BD in youth (and the potential diagnostic instability in a significant subgroup of early-onset BD cases), it is probably premature to set up diagnosis-specific, early-detection teams for BD. It is more likely that cost-effective interventions can be provided by including clinicians with specialist skills and expertise in BD within the available EIP or youth mental health service models. Given the rates of depression in youth, screening and monitoring programmes for those individuals at above-average risk of BD will probably need to operate at the interface between primary and secondary care services [18]. These service options can be revisited if BAR criteria are further refined, and possibly combined with UHR for psychosis to enhance the prediction of future illness trajectories across diagnostic boundaries [17, 25, 33].

A review of current data on interventions for individuals with emerging BD identifies that the available treatment protocols lack consideration of individual needs or unique prognostic indicators [4, 18]. A significant challenge is to develop more valid, evidence-based, timely pharmacotherapies and psychological interventions that are appropriate for different stages of BD. These developments might extend to transdiagnostic approaches to determine whether generic medications with a favourable benefit-to-risk profile, such as neuroprotective agents (e.g. antioxidants, fish oils), are effective in delaying transitions or preventing illness progression, or to explore if modifications to currently prescribed disorder-specific treatments of BD are preferable (e.g. low-dose lithium). Such advances may have implications for how we treat episodes of depression in young people who may be at risk of future bipolarity, to ensure that the most beneficial interventions for an early-onset depressive disorder do not inadvertently expose an underlying risk of BD, or accelerate transition to BD.

References

1. **Merikangas KR, Jin R, He JP, Kessler RC, Lee S, Sampson NA**, et al. Prevalence and correlates of bipolar spectrum disorder in the world mental health survey initiative. Arch Gen Psychiatry. 2011; **68**:241–51.
2. **Jones PB.** Adult mental health disorders and their age at onset. Br J Psychiatry. 2013; **202**(s54):s5–10.
3. **Gore F, Bloem P, Patton G, Ferguson J, Joseph V, Coffey C**, et al. Global burden of disease in young people aged 10–24 years: a systematic analysis. Lancet. 2011 Jun; **377**(9783):2093–102.
4. **Power P, Conus P, Macneil C, Scott J.** Early intervention in bipolar disorders. In: **Byrne P, Rosen A**, editors. Early intervention in psychiatry: EI of nearly everything for better mental health. Chichester: John Wiley; 2014. p. 432.
5. **Kupka R, Hilligers M, Scott J.** Staging systems in bipolar disorder. In: **Kapczinski F, Vieta E, Magalhaes P, Berk M**, editors. Neuroprogression and staging in bipolar disorder. Oxford: Oxford University Press; 2015. p. 344.
6. **Carlson GA, Glovinsky I.** The concept of bipolar disorder in children: a history of the bipolar controversy. Child Adolesc Psychiatr Clin N Am. 2009 Apr; **18**(2):257–71.
7. **Moreno C, Laje G, Blanco C, Jiang H, Schmidt AB, Olfson M.** National trends in the outpatient diagnosis and treatment of bipolar disorder in youth. Arch Gen Psychiatry. 2007; **64**:1032–9.
8. **Douglas J, Scott J.** Mania in pre-pubertal children: fact or artefact? Bipolar Disord. 2014; **16**(1):5–15.
9. **James A, Hoang U, Seagroatt V, Clacey J, Goldacre M, Leibenluft E.** A comparison of American and English hospital discharge rates for pediatric bipolar disorder, 2000 to 2010. J Am Acad Child Adolesc Psychiatry. 2014; **53**(6):614–24.
10. **Scott J.** Bipolar disorder: from early intervention to personalized treatment. Early Interv Psychiatry. 2011; **5**:89–90.
11. **McGorry PD, Hickie IB, Yung A, Pantelis C, Jackson H.** Clinical staging of psychiatric disorders: a heuristic framework for choosing earlier, safer and more effective interventions. Aust NZ J Psychiatry. 2006; **40**(8):616–22.
12. **Berk M, Conus P, Lucas N, Hallam K, Malhi G, Dodd S**, et al. Setting the stage: from prodrome to treatment resistance in bipolar disorder. Bipolar Disord. 2007 Nov; **9**(7):671–8.
13. **Duffy A, Alda M, Hajek T, Sherry SB, Grof P.** Early stages in the development of bipolar disorder. J Affect Disord. 2010; **121**(1–2):127–35.
14. **Hickie IB, Scott J, McGorry PD.** Clinical staging for mental disorders: a new development in diagnostic practice in mental health. Med J Aust. 2013 May 20; **198**(9):461–2.
15. **Scott J, Leboyer M, Hickie I, Berk M, Kapzinsky F, Frank E**, et al. Clinical staging in psychiatry: a cross-cutting model of diagnosis with heuristic and practical value. Br J Psychiatry. 2013 Apr; **202**(4):243–5.
16. **Kapczinski F, Magalhaes P, Balanza-Martinez V, Dias V, Frangou S, Gama C**, et al. Staging systems in bipolar disorder: an International Society for Bipolar Disorders Task Force Report. Acta Psychiatr Scand. 2014 Nov; **130**(5):354–63.

17. **Scott J, Henry C.** Clinical staging models: from general medicine to mental disorders. BJPsych Advances. 2017; **23**(5):292–9.
18. **Scott J, Scott E, Hermens D, Naismith S, Guastella A, White D,** et al. Functional impairment in adolescents and young adults with emerging mood disorders. Br J Psychiatry. 2014 Nov; **205**(5):362–8.
19. **McGorry PD, Killackey E, Yung A.** Early intervention in psychosis: concepts, evidence and future directions. World Psychiatry. 2008 Oct; 7(3):148–56.
20. **Scott J.** Early intervention in bipolar disorders. Early Interv Psychiatry. 2014; **8**(S1):28–9.
21. **Marshall M, Lewis S, Lockwood A, Drake R, Jones P, Croudace T.** Association between duration of untreated psychosis and outcome in cohorts of first-episode patients: a systematic review. Arch Gen Psychiatry. 2005; **62**:975–83.
22. **Drancourt N, Etain B, Lajnef M, Henry C, Raust A, Cochet B,** et al. Duration of untreated bipolar disorder: missed opportunities on the long road to optimal treatment. Acta Psychiatr Scand. 2013 Feb; **127**(2):136–44.
23. **Carvalho A, Takwoingi Y, Sales P, Soczynska J, Kohler C, Freitas T,** et al. Screening for bipolar spectrum disorders: a comprehensive meta-analysis of accuracy studies. J Affect Disord. 2015 Feb 1; **172**:337–46.
24. **Waugh M, Meyer T, Youngstrom E, Scott J.** A review of self-rating instruments to identify young people at risk of bipolar spectrum disorders. J Affect Disord. 2014 May; **160**:113–21.
25. **Scott J, Marwaha S, Ratheesh A, Macmillan I, Yung AR, Morriss R,** et al. Bipolar at-risk criteria: an examination of which clinical features have optimal utility for identifying youth at risk of early transition from depression to bipolar disorders. Schizophr Bull. 2016 Nov 21; **pii**:sbw154. [Epub ahead of print].
26. **Kim-Cohen J, Caspi A, Moffitt TE, Harrington H, Milne BJ, Poulton R.** Prior juvenile diagnoses in adults with mental disorder: developmental follow-back of a prospective-longitudinal cohort. Arch Gen Psychiatry. 2003 Jul; **60**(7):709–17.
27. **Loftus J, Etain B, Scott J.** What can we learn from offspring studies in bipolar disorder? BJPsych Advances. 2016; **22**(3):176–85.
28. **National Institute of Healthcare and Clinical Excellence** (NICE). Bipolar disorder (update): the management of bipolar disorder in adults, children and adolescents in primary and secondary care. London: NICE; 2014 (CG185).
29. **Correll C, Olvet D, Auther A, Hauser M, Kishimoto T, Carrion R,** et al. The Bipolar Prodrome Symptom Interview and Scale-Prospective (BPSS-P): description and validation in a psychiatric sample and healthy controls. Bipolar Disord. 2014 Aug; **16**(5):505–22.
30. **Faedda G, Marangoni C, Serra G, Salvatore P, Sani G, Vazquez G,** et al. Precursors of bipolar disorders: a systematic literature review of prospective studies. J Clin Psychiatry. 2015 May; **76**(5):614–24.
31. **Geoffroy P, Scott J.** What's in a name: prodromes and risk syndromes in bipolar disorders. Int J Bipolar Disord. 2017; **5**:7.
32. **Bechdolf A, Nelson B, Cotton SM, Chanen A, Thompson A, Kettle J,** et al. A preliminary evaluation of the validity of at-risk criteria for bipolar disorders in help-seeking adolescents and young adults. J Affect Disord. 2010; **127**:316–20.

33. **Bechdolf A, Ratheesh A, Cotton SM, Nelson B, Chanen AM, Betts J**, et al. The predictive validity of bipolar at-risk (prodromal) criteria in help-seeking adolescents and young adults: a prospective study. Bipolar Disord. 2014 Aug; **16**(5):493–504.
34. **Mitchell A.** Sensitivity×PPV is a recognized test called the clinical utility index. Eur J Epidemiol. 2011; **26**:251–2.
35. **Davidson J, Scott J.** Should we intervene at stage 0? A qualitative study of attitudes of asymptomatic youth at risk of bipolar disorders and parents with established disease. Early Interv Psychiatry. 2018 Dec; **12**(6): 1112–19.
36. **Vallarino M, Henry C, Etain B, Gehue L, Macneil C, Scott E**, et al. An evidence map of psychosocial interventions for the earliest stages of bipolar disorder. Lancet Psychiatry. 2015; **2**(6):548–63.
37. **Scott J, Hickie I, McGorry P.** Invited editorial. Pre-emptive psychiatric treatments: pipe dream or a realistic outcome of clinical staging models? Neuropsychiatry. 2012; **2**(4):263–5.
38. **Conus P, McGorry P.** First episode mania: a neglected priority for early intervention. Aust NZ J Psychiatry. 2002; **36**: 158–72.

Chapter 13

Early intervention in bipolar disorders

Setting the stage from mechanisms to models

Gin S. Malhi, Grace Morris, Amber Hamilton, and Tim Outhred

Introduction

In the majority of patients, the diagnosis and treatment of bipolar disorder (BD) is delayed, sometimes by up to a decade [1]. Hence the need to reliably detect and manage this debilitating illness much earlier is clear, and the concept of early intervention is necessarily seductive. But is it well-founded? In order for early intervention to effect change that leads to meaningful outcomes, a number of important conditions need to be met. Firstly, the disease process that one is trying to treat or prevent needs to be understood, preferably fully or at least in part, and certainly sufficiently so that any treatment or intervention is both logical and targeted. Secondly, it is important to have established that the intervention is indeed effective in achieving the desired outcome—be that immediate resolution of symptoms, the maintenance of well-being, or the prevention of future illness. Finally, such interventions should provide reasonable benefits and come at minimal cost, which requires knowledge of the long-term effects and potential damage any intervention may cause. In this chapter, we have attempted to address some of these key prerequisites for any potential early intervention strategies that may be applied to BD, and discuss those findings that have been useful, or may provide useful leads for future research.

Defining bipolar disorder

A fundamental problem when considering BD and its treatment is that its definition varies according to context. The older term 'manic-depressive illness' [2] is often mistakenly considered to be synonymous with BD, but in fact the two terms themselves are almost poles apart. The key feature of manic-depression is *recurrence*, whereas in BD the emphasis is applied to *polarity* of mood.

Interestingly, modern-day BD has also gradually drifted further away from its original foundations, adopting a spectrum model and choosing to anchor itself amongst less severe presentations. Consequently, the definitions of bipolar I and bipolar II, first introduced more than a quarter of a century ago, are nowadays seldom used as originally intended [3].

Today's view of BD is that of a heterogeneous group of illnesses spanning a spectrum comprising all manner of mood perturbations [4–6]. In this context, there has been a recent resurgence of interest in mixed states [7–9] and the overlap of mood disorder with other key sets of features such as anxiety and psychosis [6], and the predilection for substance misuse that often co-occurs [10, 11]. Even the definition of BD on the basis of manic symptoms, which distinguish mood presentations from those that feature solely as recurrent depressive symptoms, has become increasingly difficult. This confusion is primarily due to a lack of agreement regarding which symptoms signal mania, what number of symptoms are required, and for what duration they should be present before a definitive diagnosis of BD can be made (e.g. [12, 13]). Recent debates and criticisms of definitions of BD and mixed-mood states highlight all of these problems, and challenge the fundamental model of depressive and bipolar disorders, which has been wedded to giving primacy to mood and examining cross-sectional status versus longitudinal history [8, 14].

Thus, the diagnosis of BD remains a topic of debate. However, a precise definition is a necessary prerequisite for the development of early intervention strategies. Hence, we have proposed the re-introduction of the original definitions of pure mood and mixed states, along with key symptoms, in order to increase the specificity of the classification of mood disorder episodes and the identification of emergence of symptoms in established disorders [14] (see Table 13.1). The reintroduction of these signs and symptoms may allow for more accurate detection of mood disorders as symptoms heralding the emergence of the illness first manifest early in its course.

All of the complexities with delineating BD are magnified when considering the diagnosis of BD in youth, especially in adolescence or even younger still in children [15]. Consequently, the diagnosis of paediatric BD varies hugely both in terms of the definitions used and reported prevalence [16]. It remains unclear which symptoms are key to the diagnosis of mania and whether these remain the same in youth, adolescents, and children [17]. Given the neurodevelopmental changes that occur within the brain and the degree of maturation needed for the expression of symptoms [18], it is highly unlikely that the definitions can be the same across different epochs of early life. Perhaps until BD can be defined with confidence in children and adolescents, it would be prudent to adopt a more conservative approach and set the threshold for diagnosis relatively high. For example, adopting a 'narrow' definition would mean that a firm diagnosis

Table 13.1 More specific classification of mood disorder states (based on Weygandt's conceptualization), which may prove more useful for earlier detection than the current classificatory systems

Mood state	Mood	Thought	Activity
Pure			
1. Depressive	–	–	–
2. Manic	+	+	+
Mixed			
3. Depressive mania (irritable mania)	–	+	+
4. Depressive excitement	–	–	+
5. Depression with flight of ideas	–	+	–
6. Manic stupor	+	–	–
7. Depression with flight of ideas and emotional elations (inhibited mania)	+	+	–
8. Unproductive mania	+	–	+

Key: + = activated; – = inhibited

Set of symptoms to be considered: manic symptoms (in context of depression); distractibility; irritability; depressive symptoms (in context of mania); psychomotor agitation; diminished ability to think or concentrate, or indecisiveness.

Source data from: *Australian & New Zealand Journal of Psychiatry*, 50, 7, Malhi GS, Byrow Y, Fritz K., Mixed mood states: time to adopt a 3D perspective? SAGE Publications 2016; *Bipolar Disorders*, 19, 4, Malhi GS, Berk M, Morris G, Hamilton A, Outhred T, Das P, et al., Mixed Mood: The not so united states? 2017, John Wiley and Sons.

could only be made when symptoms akin to those characterizing the illness in adults are clearly evident. This would allow the early signs and symptoms of adult-type BD to be traced. At the same time, broader and alternative definitions could be researched to better understand how individual symptoms emerge and coalesce to form BD.

Determinants of treatment

Timing: determining when to treat

As in many things in life, when considering the treatment of BD 'timing is everything'. Even in cases where the emergence of BD is inevitable, intervention can be commenced at various stages of the illness—from when the diagnosis is absolutely *confirmed* to when it is likely (e.g. on the basis of an initial depressive episode a diagnosis is not yet established but *probable*). Interventions can also be commenced further back still, to a period of time when the diagnosis is *possible* on the basis of risk factors for BD and emerging transient signs and symptoms (see Fig. 13.1). However, mapping any such steps and reliably differentiating

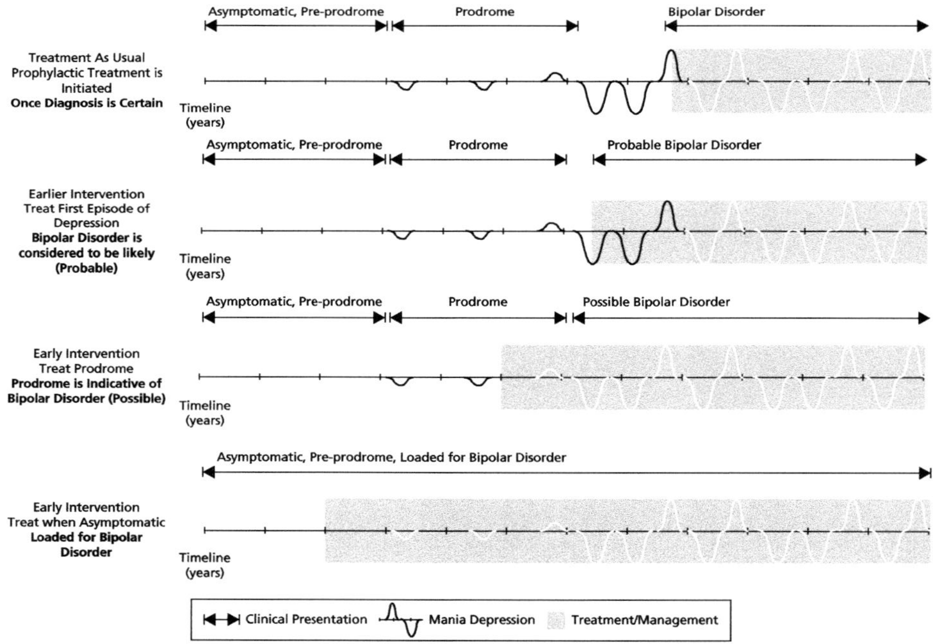

Fig. 13.1 Timing of early intervention in bipolar disorder: early or earlier? Early intervention is predicated on the assumption that bipolar disorder will occur and that the intervention will confer prophylaxis. A critical problem is the natural history of bipolar disorder because it typically presents with depressive symptoms that are essentially indistinguishable from major depressive disorder. The latter is generally more common and usually requires different management strategies. Therefore, if the first episode is depressive and considered to be the beginning of a bipolar illness, prophylactic treatment given at this time may be regarded as early intervention—preventing the emergence of mania. Early intervention thus consists of administering prophylactic treatment once a prodrome has been established, at the first sign of the prodrome, or even prior, when asymptomatic. The schematic shows where intervention that has prophylactic effects commences. It is described as various kinds of early intervention, depending on when it is instituted.

them solely on the basis of the phenomenology of BD, the majority of which is non-specific and often transient, is near impossible. Furthermore, without definitive biomarkers that predict BD, the current reality is that early intervention is reliant on the emergence of initial symptoms, at which point 'early' intervention is probably already too late (not early enough). This is because clinical symptoms are the culmination of underlying changes and processes within the brain that eventually lead to the expression of full-blown BD. Thus clinically, although there is a strong and understandable desire to intervene as early as possible, in the nascent stages of BD it is unclear whether initial fluctuations in symptomatology will actually develop into sustained changes that characterize the illness.

It is important to recognize that in most cases early intervention is simply 'earlier intervention'. That is to say, it is the same treatment essentially being administered 'earlier', rather than a separate set of treatments designed specifically to have a prophylactic effect. Indeed, currently such novel treatments are not available, and what precisely they would change also remains a matter for conjecture. In practice, there are no definitive 'tests' to diagnose BD and no means to objectively determine prognosis—thus at present, early intervention is more of a goal than a reality. The best prognostic data available at the moment is that classification from major depressive disorder (MDD) to BD is most likely to occur within five years, but only a small proportion of cases make the transition [19]. Over a 12-year period, less than 25 per cent of MDD cases transition to BD [19]. Therefore, early intervention in BD needs to be considered with cautious enthusiasm, and a delicate balance needs to be maintained. For example, extremely early intervention could result in treating individuals who would have only experienced transient symptomatology that would have resolved of its own accord; at the same time, waiting for symptoms to coalesce into syndromes before intervening could mean an important window of opportunity for treatment is missed. This tension, as well as the lack of knowledge regarding the benefits and risks of interventions at different stages, which informs the decision as to when to intervene, has meant that the early intervention paradigm in BD remains poorly defined and unsubstantiated by research.

Treatment specificity

The treatment of BD is equally as problematic as its diagnosis, prognostication, and treatment timing. The question of specificity can also be linked to diagnosis, such that pharmacotherapeutic interventions could target specific phases of the illness and only be trialled in patients that clearly meet stringent criteria for mania—specifically, heightened energy and activity along with cognitive change, with equal emphasis on these domains alongside changes in mood.

Other than lithium, no treatment has been developed specifically for the treatment of manic depression—the forerunner of bipolarity [20]. All remaining agents currently in use have migrated from other fields after having been trialled optimistically in the treatment of all aspects of BD. Predictably, these have had variable success [21]. The main problem is that of specificity (i.e. the administration of treatments specifically for BD), which is inherently linked to the difficulties of accurate and reliable diagnosis and the lack of knowledge regarding the underlying pathophysiology of the illness [22]. Empirically, even in patients with BD who are well characterized and have a clear pattern of recurrent mood episodes that are recognizable and discrete, with significant periods of remission in between, the effectiveness of lithium is significantly less than half [23]. In practice, probably only a third of patients respond well and maintain wellness on lithium when characterized clinically as 'potential lithium responders' [23]. Nevertheless, compared to the other treatments currently available, the effectiveness of lithium for BD is impressive, and at least it provides a starting point from which it may be possible to build a systematic approach to testing treatments. For example, by targeting those individuals likely to respond to lithium and identifying lithium responders, the remaining individuals (lithium non-responders) can then be tested separately for their response to other treatments [24]. Akin to what occurs in oncology (where treatment response greatly informs diagnosis and prognosis), identifying lithium non-responders at the onset creates a slightly more homogenous population (with respect to treatment responsivity) for further investigation (see Fig. 13.2). By carving BD in this way [24], its treatment profile can be more specific, and its biology may be better understood, perhaps facilitating earlier detection of the illness.

It is clear that therapeutic development is essential for early intervention for BD. Potential lithium mimetics such as Ebselen [25] and future development of novel mood stabilizers [26] may prove useful for the treatment of both the full-blown disorder and earlier intervention. Even if these future mood-stabilizer medications are less effective than lithium itself for fully established bipolar disorder, they may prove useful to attenuate the early signs of the disorder or to reduce the severity or frequency of episodes during the course of a potential bipolar illness, particularly if they are safer to administer and are better tolerated. In this manner, additional interventions that are designed for emergent symptoms and are more targeted towards milder symptoms could allow for a combination of treatment strategies (early intervention and 'wait and see'), at least until illness characteristics become definitive, at which point interventions can be escalated or withdrawn accordingly.

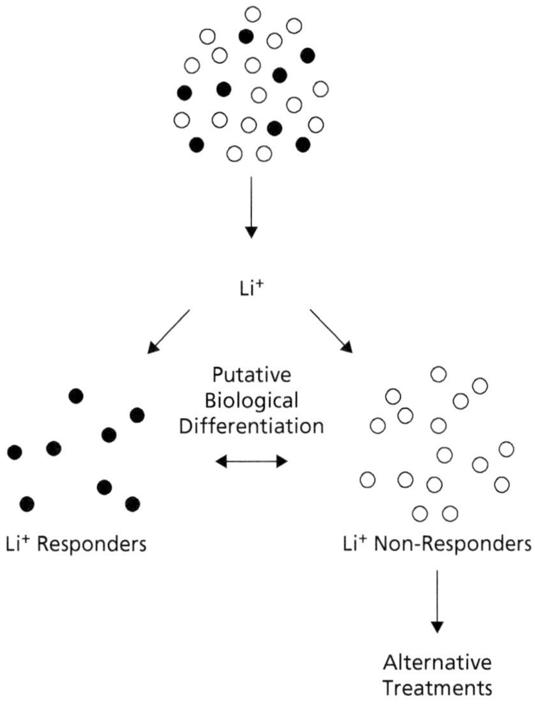

Fig. 13.2 Carving bipolarity using a lithium sword.

Mechanisms and models

Aetiology: where to begin

The precise aetiology of BD is unknown; however, both genetic and environmental factors have been linked with the development of early-onset BD [27]. Family studies have revealed that having an immediate family member with a mood disorder increases the risk of developing BD compared to the general population [28, 29]. It is important to note that while there is high heritability for BD, not all offspring of BD parents will develop a psychiatric disorder [30]. Stressful life events and psychosocial stress also play an important role in the onset and course of BD. Additional risk factors include childhood sexual abuse and trauma, which have both been associated with earlier onset and higher severity of illness for BD [31]. Also noteworthy is the fact that substance use and BD commonly co-occur [11, 32], although as of yet it is uncertain whether substance use produces symptoms that resemble BD symptoms or whether substance use precipitates BD symptoms in vulnerable individuals [11].

Importantly, the classification of BD is not derived from aetiology; rather, it remains tied to psychopathology and clinical phenomenology. That is to say, diagnosis is generally based on risk factors, course of illness, and individual's response to treatment. A diagnosis of BD can, therefore, be derived from a variety of pathophysiological processes and, while the manifestation of symptom presentation may appear similar between individuals and across populations, the actual aetiology could be very different. Thus, linking aetiology to diagnosis is likely to be even more complicated when attempting to do so in the context of early detection and intervention. As an initial attempt to navigate these issues, staging models have been proposed.

Staging models are routinely used in general medicine for chronic physical disorders (e.g. oncology) to provide a framework for links between biomarkers, clinical phenotypes, and disease progression, with a view to inform treatment. By virtue of the chronic and progressive nature of BD, clinical staging models have become increasingly popular for mapping neuroprogression. However, staging models are predicated on the assumption that an individual can be accurately positioned along a continuum that represents the illness course. This point can then provide insight into stage-appropriate interventions and treatments. A number of proposed clinical staging models (see Table 13.2) for BD categorize different stages of illness, ranging from *Stage 0* (an individual has an increased risk of BD based on psychosocial and genetic factors, but there is an absence of any identifiable symptoms) to *Stage 4* (an individual has a severe, persistent, and

Table 13.2 A proposed clinical staging model for bipolar disorder

Clinical stage	Definition of stages
Stage 0	Increased risk of severe mood disorder (e.g. family history, abuse, substance use). No specific symptoms.
Stage 1	(a) Mild or non-specific symptoms of mood disorder. (b) Prodromal features—ultra-high risk: moderate but subthreshold symptoms.
Stage 2	First episode of mood disorder. Threshold disorder with moderate to severe symptoms, neurocognitive deficits, and functional decline.
Stage 3	(a) Recurrence of subthreshold mood symptoms—incomplete remission from first episode. (b) First threshold relapse. (c) Multiple relapses.
Stage 4	Persistent unremitting illness.

Adapted from *Bipolar disorders*, 9, 7, Berk M, Conus P, Lucas N, Hallam K, Malhi GS, Dodd S, et al., Setting the stage: from prodrome to treatment resistance in bipolar disorder, pp. 671–678.

unremitting illness) [33–35]. Currently, the understanding of Stage 4 in terms of diagnosis and treatment outcomes greatly outweighs the knowledge of the prodromal phase (pre-diagnosis/high-risk phase). Theoretically, a staging model should provide a useful algorithm to identify at-risk periods and offer a platform for implementing stage-appropriate treatments during the early stages of the illness, to curb its progression and enhance the chances of recovery.

A staging model that maps BD has the potential to guide treatment and prognosis while providing a framework for further investigation of the disease. However, the evidence to support such a universal staging structure is lacking due to various methodological limitations [36]. For example, there is a paucity of longitudinal studies of psychopathology and biomarkers in genetically at-risk individuals [37]. Consequently, there is a need for longitudinal studies investigating well-defined subgroups of genetic and clinically high-risk youths, to enable the mapping of biomarkers onto emerging psychopathology, before a valid and meaningful staging model can be developed [38].

Evolution and development

There is often a substantial delay, which can be up to five to ten years, between the onset of first symptoms and diagnosis of BD [1, 39]. Correctly identifying BD in its early stages is a challenge as the substantial emotional, social, and cognitive development that occurs during adolescence and early adulthood can both mask and be misinterpreted as bipolar symptomatology. This developmental phase naturally obscures the initial identification and diagnosis of BD [15].

The escalating impetus for early intervention strategies has led to the desire to identify particular precursors to developing BD. Early symptoms that are distinct from normality but do not yet express the psychopathology of BD have been described putatively as a *prodrome* [40]. The prodromal phase of BD refers to the time from the initial onset of signs and symptoms to the diagnosis of BD [40]. According to the staging model, the prodromal phase spans Stage 0 and Stage 1 (see Table 13.2). The concept of a prodrome provides a potentially useful foundation for understanding the evolution and development of BD. It is proposed that the prodromal phase can be subdivided into three components [41]. First, the *pre-prodromal period* refers to the underlying pathophysiological processes which have not yet reached the tipping point and emerged as symptoms. Second, the *distal prodrome* denotes the early stages of symptoms emerging, generally in adolescents. Third, the *proximal prodrome* encompasses the later end of the prodromal phase, commonly in early adulthood and immediately prior to the emergence of the first episode of BD (depressive or manic).

Early intervention strategies for progressive psychiatric illnesses rely on the identification and presentation of a disorder prodrome. Thus, it is concerning that the evidence in support of the presence of a bipolar prodrome is extremely mixed. In a review of the literature investigating the bipolar prodrome, it was revealed that 28 studies identified mood lability, depressive mood, and irritability as the most cited prodromal features [41]. The same review also revealed large methodological flaws in the research conducted in this area, including recall bias in retrospective studies, inconsistencies of the operationalization of the prodromal phase, a lack of comparison groups, and a lack of generalizability.

Along with methodological issues, the absence of quality research investigating the bipolar prodrome can be traced to a number of compounding factors. First, the natural course of BD often begins with episodes of depression, meaning that it regularly goes undiagnosed as major depression until manic episodes or mixed states appear [12]. Secondly, it is extremely difficult to disaggregate a bipolar prodrome from natural developmental changes that take place over the course of childhood and adolescence [15]. For example, stress, impulsivity, and mood and emotional lability could be misinterpreted as preclinical signs. Furthermore, not all individuals undergo a prodromal period, as some can experience immediate onset of a BD episode and have a full manifestation of the illness without first being subjected to milder symptoms [42].

Clearly, BD is a complex recurrent illness characterized by innumerable co-morbidities, presentations, and phases [43], and, at this 'stage' of nascent knowledge, it does not seem feasible to accurately identify individuals who may develop BD purely based on the identification of a prodrome consisting of early signs and symptoms.

Bipolar brain biology

Since the development of functional neuroimaging, researchers have looked to identify the brain structures and neurocognitive processes that underpin BD. However, despite significant advancements in imaging technology, studies have revealed that the biology of the brain in BD is deeply complex and that episodes of mania and depression produce widespread changes in the brain, rather than simply affecting particular regions [44]. Nevertheless, such research has identified significant differences in the brain structures of people with BD compared to healthy controls. For example, Strakowski and colleagues [45], and others more recently [46], observed volumetric differences in the neural structures, such as enlargement of the amygdala which is associated with emotional expression and stimulus-reward learning and, therefore, implicated in the regulation of mood. Such studies indicate that there may be significant differences in the brain structures of patients with BD and healthy populations. An understanding of these differences would be invaluable in identifying populations at risk of BD and developing targeted treatment interventions. However, at present, the research findings are inconsistent and it is unknown to what extent these brain changes pre-empt the disorder, are caused by the disorder, or are iatrogenically caused by psychotropic medications [47].

Through the use of functional neuroimaging, other researchers have sought to develop models of the dysfunctional neural mechanisms that may drive BD [48–52]. Although nuanced, many of these models give primacy to the cognitive processes of suppression, attentional control, reappraisal, rumination, and reward processing in the regulation of mood [53]. These cognitive processes that work to regulate emotions and modulate mood are hypothesized to be supported by a set of brain structures, depicted in Fig. 13.3. Again, it is apparent

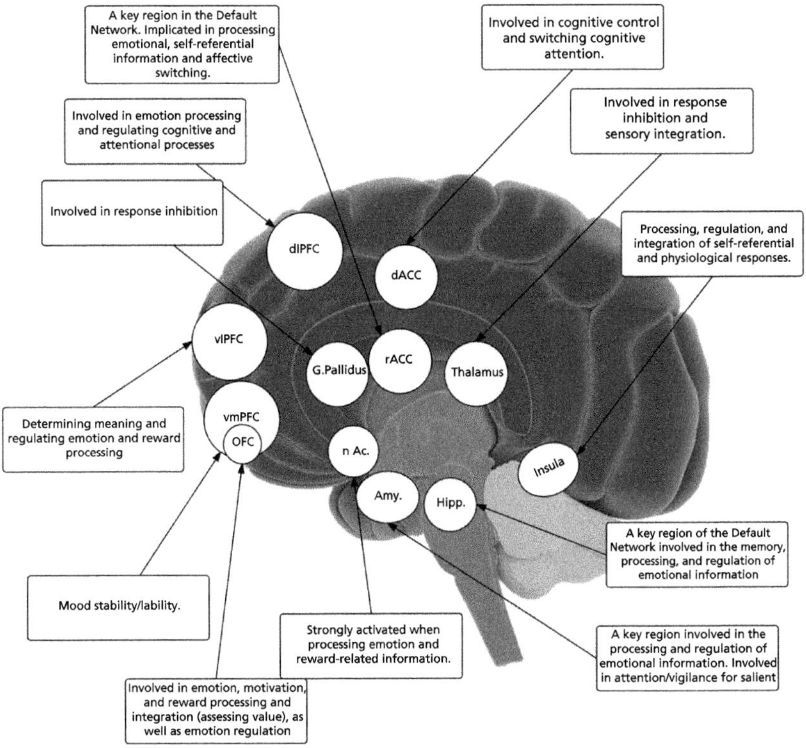

Fig. 13.3 Key brain regions implicated in mood disorders.

Key: Amy. = amygdala; dACC = dorsal anterior cingulate cortex; dlPFC = dorsolateral prefrontal cortex; G.Pallidus = globus pallidus; Hipp. = hippocampus; n.Ac. = nucleus accumbens; OFC = orbital frontal cortex; rACC = rostral anterior cingulate cortex; vlPFC = ventrolateral prefrontal cortex; vmPFC = ventromedial prefrontal cortex.

Reproduced from *Bipolar Disorders*, 17, S2, Malhi GS, Byrow Y, Fritz K, Das P, Baune BT, Porter RJ, et al, Mood disorders: neurocognitive models, pp. 3–20. Copyright (2015) with permission from John Wiley and Sons.

that the neurocognitive processes involved in the modulations of mood in BD involve global brain networks and cannot be fully explained by perturbations in a single region or circuit.

Clearly, the functional psychophysiology of BD is complicated and, to a great extent, remains unknown. Notably, research has not yet uncovered a dysfunctional brain structure or process that has specificity in predicting the onset and course of BD, a prognostic insight that would be invaluable in identifying prodromal bipolarity [41]. Nevertheless, it is important that research continues to integrate our current understanding of the volumetric changes in brain structure with the functional cognitive processes that underpin mood perturbations as well as our knowledge of endocrine systems, and neurotransmitter and synaptic alterations, in order to gain a deeper and more complete understanding of BD brain pathophysiology. Only the latter can inform treatment and facilitate the detection of suitable target populations putatively responsive to early intervention.

Mechanisms of mood

There are three central components of mood disorders—emotion, cognition, and behaviour [54]—that can be examined against the backdrop of neurocognitive models so as to provide a greater understanding of the mechanisms of mood disorders. A synthesis and critical analysis of extant models of neurocognition in mood disorders [53] shows that a number of dysfunctional cognitive processes underpin mood disorders. First, patients with mood disorders have shown a decreased and less successful use of *reappraisal* strategies when processing negative cognitions, suggesting that reappraisal may play an important role in the development, maintenance, and treatment of depressive symptoms [48, 55]. Second, *rumination* is maladaptive among patients with BD and has been shown to be linked to depressive symptom severity [56]. Third, dysfunctional *attention deployment and control* may be a risk factor for developing a mood disorder as extended processing of negative information compromises emotion-regulation strategies [57]. Fourth, irregular *reward processing* in patients with BD is associated with deficits in decision making (e.g. impulsivity, emotional processing, high risk taking, and high reward choices [58]).

As previously discussed, *DSM-5*'s phenomenology-based diagnosis does not allow for early detection of mood disorders. Therefore, the knowledge gained by the further investigation of these neurocognitive deficits may provide a framework to examine and potentially identify differences in neurobiological markers underlying mood disorders. In particular, using neuroimaging to tease apart MDD and BD diagnoses could help identify distinct biomarkers for each disorder. For example, dysfunctional processing within the amygdala is associated with both BD and MDD; however, Grotegard and colleagues [59] investigated amygdala activation in response to emotional stimuli and found that BD participants displayed greater right-sided activation in the amygdala when presented with happy faces, whereas MDD participants exhibited greater activation in the amygdala when presented with sad faces. Similarly, BD patients can be distinguished from MDD patients through the interrogation of reward-processing impairments [60]. Consequently, identifying dysfunctional cognitive processes as neurobiological markers of mood disorder is a positive step towards our goal of accurately diagnosing BD and developing techniques for early detection. Nevertheless, additional clinically valid research is required to confirm the clinical utility of these results.

Early intervention: current pitfalls and potential rewards

In the previous sections, the limitations of our understanding of BD and the goals of early intervention were discussed in detail. In light of these, the risks, pitfalls, and potential benefits of early intervention are now considered specifically—modifying illness trajectory, containment, and prevention.

Divining trajectory

Accurately identifying BD in its early stages is a challenge because of the extensive emotional, social, and cognitive development that takes place during adolescence and early adulthood. Changes in these domains can both obscure the symptomology of BD and be misinterpreted as signs and symptoms of the illness. Thus, there is considerable risk attached to being too definitive when identifying 'prodromal' BD, because what may appear to be manic or depressive symptoms may indeed be a part of normal adolescent development [41]. This risk of over-identifying 'prodromal' stages of BD is particularly worrisome as diagnosis usually begets treatment, which might culminate in the premature administration of psychotropic medications that may affect illness trajectory.

As previously mentioned, the mapping of the natural course of BD and illness progression onto a clinical staging model has been attempted; however, BD is a lifelong, capricious illness with a myriad of patterns and variations in course [43]. Hence, intervention strategies and the call for earlier treatment administration is particularly concerning, especially as it is currently unknown whether premature psychotropic medication may actually worsen the course of BD. Emerging research has recommended different types of interventions for different stages of illness. For example, McGorry and colleagues [61] propose that there may be some utility in providing psychoeducation and cognitive behaviour therapy (CBT), encouraging substance use reduction as well as administering atypical antipsychotics, antidepressants, or mood stabilizers for those who are identified as being 'ultra-high risk' of developing BD. Similarly, McNamara and colleagues [62] recommend that lighter interventions, such as dietary and psychosocial interventions, should take primacy in the early stages of illness; however, if these do not improve symptoms, then these at-risk populations should be given medications.

Interestingly, although early interventions involving pharmacotherapy are tentatively recommended in the literature, there is a paucity of empirical evidence supporting their use for prodromal BD, especially amongst children and adolescents. This is particularly problematic as the first signs and symptoms of BD tend to emerge in childhood, adolescence, or early adulthood [15]. Furthermore, although the use of mood stabilizers such as lithium, valproate, carbamazepine, and atypical antipsychotics is supported by the Treatment Guidelines for Children and Adolescents with Bipolar Disorder [63], concurrent research suggests that these medications may not be efficacious for younger populations. For example, Kowatch and colleagues [64] tested the efficacy of lithium and valproate in children aged 8 to 18 and found that for more than half the children, monotherapy with either of these agents yielded no improvement in bipolar symptomatology. In fact, Kowatch and colleagues [64] observed that valproate, which has efficacy in managing BD in adults, actually exacerbated BD symptoms in children after three weeks, suggesting that the effectiveness of mood-stabilizing medications may differ substantially according to patients' developmental stage. In a similar vein, Findling and colleagues [65] observed that valproate was not superior to placebo in treating adolescents deemed to be 'at-risk' of BD. These findings are noteworthy, as they reveal that the pharmacotherapies being touted as effective 'early interventions' may, in fact, be inappropriate for the age group and phase of illness they are targeting. These findings call for more rigorous research to investigate the efficacy of medications on the early symptoms of BD that present in younger populations.

Psychotropic medications are also associated with severe adverse side-effects, such as metabolic consequences (i.e. weight gain and diabetes), risk of polycystic ovarian syndrome, and extrapyramidal symptoms [21]. Without a strong evidence base for prescribing these medications for early stages of BD, young patients could be exposed to these adverse side-effects without any clear benefit to their illness course. Of particular concern is the fact that little is known about the effects of psychotropic medications and polypharmacy on the developing brain [66]. During adolescence and early adulthood, the brain is undergoing a process of significant change as synapses are continually being remodelled and pruned [67]. As prodromal BD is most likely to be identified in adolescence, it is imperative that rigorous research is conducted to investigate the effects of psychotropic medication on executive functioning, decision making, and other critical cognitive and emotional processes during such a vulnerable time of brain development. By prematurely prescribing these medications, without first thoroughly investigating the consequences, we may be inadvertently accelerating the progress of the illness, and making individuals more vulnerable to the development of other psychiatric disorders. Therefore, although early intervention aims to improve illness course, at present the prospect lacks empirical support. Instead, the administration of psychotropic medication to vulnerable populations, in addition to being ineffective, may in fact exacerbate matters.

Curing versus containing a moving target

Staging models and their respective interventions are predicated on the assumption that the interventions for the earlier phases of illness yield a better response from patients and are more benign compared to the more invasive and less effective treatments in the latter phases [22]. In illnesses such as cancer, this model may be accurate, as the earlier interventions are less invasive and rigorous, and usually result in better outcomes for patients [22]. However, for psychiatric illnesses such as BD, this issue is more complex. For instance, although Berk and colleagues [68] found evidence to suggest that 'early-stage' individuals had a more favourable response to atypical antipsychotics compared to patients who had experienced more illness episodes, these participants still went on to experience further episodes (relapse). Findings such as these indicate that earlier intervention with medication is not a cure, but perhaps merely a method of containing the early symptoms of BD and defining the emergence of illness. Interestingly, the therapies used in early intervention have been devised for the prophylactic management of established BD and not as preventative or curative treatments when the illness is nascent. Thus, it may be futile to expect that implementing these same interventions earlier in the illness course would result in a 'cure', and the primary goal of early intervention in today's practice should be to prevent the transmutation of high-risk status into diagnosable BD [41]. However, even on this pathway there may be pitfalls.

Early intervention treatments for identified at-risk individuals also bear the risk of producing iatrogenic symptoms, which would be difficult to distinguish from gradually emerging BD symptoms. Thus, medicating emergent bipolarity may cause changes in the presentation of the illness, which then require further treatment and modification, and so on. In other words, once an intervention has been instituted, the treatment target may change. Indeed, treatment targets will likely continue to shift throughout the course of the illness, because of the nature of the disease process and also the impact of the treatment itself. Additionally, the core pathophysiological process of the illness may adapt in response to an early intervention and, in doing so, take the illness along an altogether new trajectory.

Preventing versus prolonging

The difficulty with the concept of early intervention is that it implies that by encouraging earlier treatments and therapies, we may entirely prevent the onset of illness. However, with BD, as with other psychiatric disorders, this is an unknown, as the aetiology and processes underpinning the development and progression of BD are still very much a mystery. As research is still underway to identify biomarkers and other predisposing features, we do not know yet whether BD can be prevented by such early interventions, or whether the onset of the disorder is largely inevitable [41]. If it is the latter, early intervention may in fact be extending the period of treatment that an individual undergoes during their lifetime, without any obvious benefit. In addition, early intervention may actually be encouraging individuals to engage in burdensome psychological and pharmacological interventions, before they are actually needed, which do little to prevent the onset of a severe episode.

Recommendations based on current evidence and practices

The dearth of evidence for early intervention has been clearly highlighted. Therefore, a conservative yet engaged approach is likely required. Cautious and tentative provisional diagnoses that are able to be removed can reduce the risk of mislabelling, and a stepped care plan to delay higher-risk treatments until necessary is a balanced approach that is likely to ensure optimal benefit.

Establishment of a therapeutic alliance is the single most important early intervention, and awareness—knowing the signs—and encouragement of help-seeking behaviour should always be the first step. In those at greatest risk of BD, clinicians may consider a stepped care model that aligns with the stage of illness (see Fig. 13.4). Clinicians can prioritize interventions, for example, as follows:

1) exercise, avoidance of substance misuse, and lifestyle changes;
2) bolster support and social structures (e.g. family therapy);
3) closer monitoring and mapping of mood, activity, and thinking;
4) psychotherapy to address known vulnerabilities (e.g. trauma) and at the emergence of the full-blown episode (diagnosed without doubt);
5) medical interventions, such as pharmacotherapy.

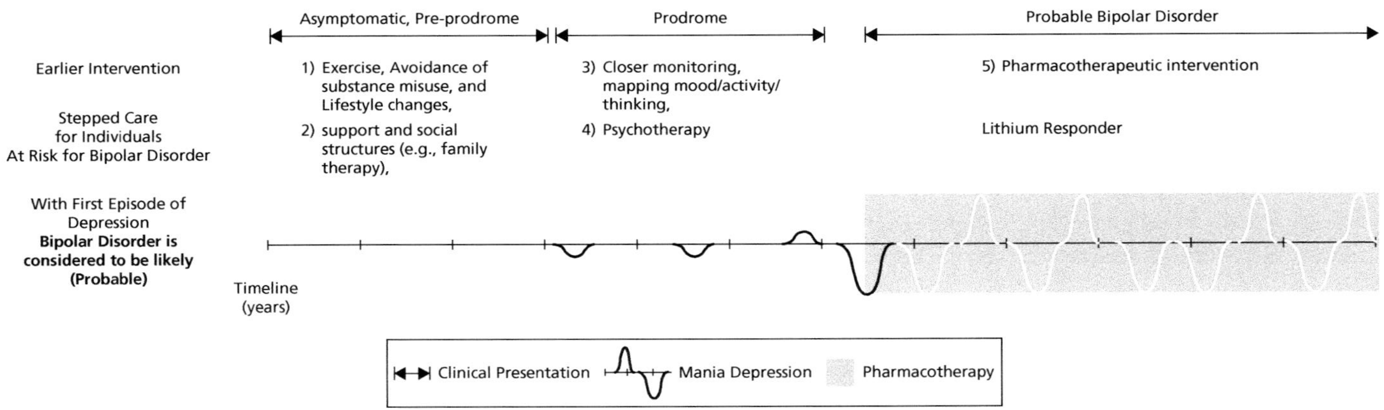

Fig. 13.4 Best-case scenario for earlier intervention in bipolar disorder based on current evidence. With the first episode of depression in patients considered to be at risk order, bipolar disorder may be considered likely. Here, the aim of earlier intervention is to prevent bipolar disorder perturbations from continuing. Management can be initiated in a stepped-care fashion, according to likely benefits balanced against the risks of treatment and no treatment.

The difficulty here is whether to adopt a depressive disorder or bipolar disorder treatment algorithm—given that in both instances, the initial presentation is most likely to be that of a depressive episode. However, as lithium therapy is indicated for both sets of disorders, it can be employed in all cases and may help identify responders early in the course of the illness. Lithium though is relatively poor in effecting significant change in acute depressive symptoms, so it would need to be used as an augmentation strategy alongside an antidepressant. Alternatively, a selective serotonin reuptake inhibitor (SSRI) could be administered, while closely monitoring for a treatment-emergent affective switch (TEAS). If this occurs, the diagnosis is likely to be BD, and the SSRI should be immediately withdrawn (for a complete discussion, see Malhi and colleagues [69]). In this way, clinicians may not need to wait until the first manic episode occurs and may be able to treat a provisional diagnosis of BD in those at greatest risk. However, there are many risks with this approach. Rather than basing prognostication and differential diagnosis on treatment response, ideally these aspects need to be determined on the basis of clinical knowledge and the use of biomarkers—tools that are yet to be developed.

Conclusions

In this chapter, we have addressed some of the key conceptual considerations for early intervention in BD. We have shown that there are currently too many gaps in our understanding of the disorder's nosology, signs, and symptoms; disease processes and progression; and intervention timing and specificity. As such, the risks of diagnosing BD within the current taxonomy and attempting to intervene early with existing treatments, which were not designed and have not been trialled for this purpose, outweigh any potential benefits. Therefore, the only recommendation for early intervention in BD we offer is to consider an initial depressive episode as a potential bipolar depressive episode and to provisionally diagnose BD on the basis of a longitudinal assessment, and then monitor and treat accordingly. Until significant progress on these numerous and highly complicated fronts is achieved, a more conservative approach for early intervention in BD is warranted.

References

1. **Lish JD, Dime-Meenan S, Whybrow PC, Price RA, Hirschfeld RM.** The National Depressive and Manic-Depressive Association (DMDA) survey of bipolar members. J Affect Disord. 1994; **31**(4):281–94.
2. **Kraepelin E.** Manic depressive insanity and paranoia. J Nerv Ment Dis. 1921; **53**(4):350.

3. **American Psychiatric Association.** DSM-IV: diagnostic and statistical manual. Washington (DC): American Psychiatric Association; 1994.
4. **Judd LL, Akiskal HS, Schettler PJ, Coryell W, Endicott J, Maser JD**, et al. A prospective investigation of the natural history of the long-term weekly symptomatic status of bipolar II disorder. Arch Gen Psychiatry. 2003; **60**(3):261–9.
5. **Judd LL, Akiskal HS, Schettler PJ, Endicott J, Maser J, Solomon DA**, et al. The long-term natural history of the weekly symptomatic status of bipolar I disorder. Arch Gen Psychiatry. 2002; **59**(6):530–7.
6. **Merikangas KR, Jin R, He J-P, Kessler RC, Lee S, Sampson NA**, et al. Prevalence and correlates of bipolar spectrum disorder in the world mental health survey initiative. Arch Gen Psychiatry. 2011; **68**(3):241–51.
7. **Fagiolini A, Coluccia A, Maina G, Forgione RN, Goracci A, Cuomo A**, et al. Diagnosis, epidemiology and management of mixed states in bipolar disorder. CNS Drugs. 2015; **29**(9):725–40.
8. **Malhi GS, Byrow Y, Fritz K.** Mixed mood states: time to adopt a 3D perspective? Aust NZ J Psychiatry; 2016; **50**(7):613–5.
9. **Malhi GS, Lampe L, Coulston CM, Tanious M, Bargh DM, Curran G**, et al. Mixed state discrimination: a DSM problem that won't go away? J Affect Disord. 2014; **158**:8–10.
10. **Di Florio A, Craddock N, Van den Bree M.** Alcohol misuse in bipolar disorder. A systematic review and meta-analysis of comorbidity rates. Eur Psychiatry. 2014; **29**(3):117–24.
11. **Strakowski SM, DelBello MP, Fleck DE, Arndt S.** The impact of substance abuse on the course of bipolar disorder. Biol Psychiatry. 2000; **48**(6):477–85.
12. **Berk M, Dodd S, Malhi GS.** 'Bipolar missed states': the diagnosis and clinical salience of bipolar mixed states. Aust NZ J Psychiatry. 2005; **39**(4):215–21.
13. **Malhi GS.** Diagnosis of bipolar disorder: who is in a mixed state? Lancet. 2013; **381**(9878):1599.
14. **Malhi GS, Berk M, Morris G, Hamilton A, Outhred T, Das P**, et al. Mixed mood: the not so united states? Bipolar Disord. 2017; **19**(4):242–5.
15. **Cahill CM, Green MJ, Jairam R, Malhi GS.** Bipolar disorder in children and adolescents: obstacles to early diagnosis and future directions. Early Interv Psychiatry. 2007; **1**(2):138–49.
16. **Biederman J, Mick E, Faraone SV, Spencer T, Wilens TE, Wozniak J.** Current concepts in the validity, diagnosis and treatment of paediatric bipolar disorder. Int J Neuropsychopharmacol. 2003; **6**(3):293–300.
17. **McClellan J, Kowatch R, Findling RL.** Practice parameter for the assessment and treatment of children and adolescents with bipolar disorder. J Am Acad Child Adolesc Psychiatry. 2007; **46**(1):107–25.
18. **Paus T, Keshavan M, Giedd JN.** Why do many psychiatric disorders emerge during adolescence? Nat Rev Neurosci. 2008; **9**(12):947–57.
19. **Ratheesh A, Davey C, Hetrick S, Alvarez-Jimenez M, Voutier C, Bechdolf A**, et al. A systematic review and meta-analysis of prospective transition from major depression to bipolar disorder. Acta Psychiatr Scand. 2017; **135**(4):273–84.
20. **Geddes JR, Miklowitz DJ.** Treatment of bipolar disorder. Lancet. 2013; **381**(9878):1672–82.

21. **Malhi GS, Bassett D, Boyce P, Bryant R, Fitzgerald PB, Fritz K,** et al. Royal Australian and New Zealand College of Psychiatrists clinical practice guidelines for mood disorders. Aust NZ J Psychiatry. 2015; **49**(12):1087–206.
22. **Malhi GS, Rosenberg DR, Gershon S.** Staging a protest! Bipolar Disord. 2014; **16**(7):776–9.
23. **Grof P.** Selecting effective long-term treatment for bipolar patients: monotherapy and combinations. J Clin Psychiatry. 2003; **64**:53–61.
24. **Malhi GS, Geddes JR.** Carving bipolarity using a lithium sword. Br J Psychiatry. 2014; **205**(5):337–9.
25. **Singh N, Halliday AC, Thomas JM, Kuznetsova OV, Baldwin R, Woon EC,** et al. A safe lithium mimetic for bipolar disorder. Nat Commun. 2013; **4**:1332.
26. **Malhi GS, Morris G, Hamilton A, Das P, Outhred T.** The ideal mood stabiliser: a quest for nirvana? Aust NZ J Psychiatry. 2017; **51**(5):434–5.
27. **Alloy LB, Abramson LY, Urosevic S, Walshaw PD, Nusslock R, Neeren AM.** The psychosocial context of bipolar disorder: environmental, cognitive, and developmental risk factors. Clin Psychol Rev. 2005; **25**(8):1043–75.
28. **Faraone SV, Glatt SJ, Tsuang MT.** The genetics of pediatric-onset bipolar disorder. Biol Psychiatry. 2003; **53**(11):970–7.
29. **Smoller JW, Finn CT.** Family, twin, and adoption studies of bipolar disorder. Am J Med Genet C Semin Med Genet. 2003; **15**; **123C**(1):48–58.
30. **Malhi GS, Moore J, McGuffin P.** The genetics of major depressive disorder. Curr Psychiatry Rep. 2000; **2**(2):165–9.
31. **Post R, Leverich G.** The role of psychosocial stress in the onset and progression of bipolar disorder and its comorbidities: the need for earlier and alternative modes of therapeutic intervention. Dev Psychopathol. 2006; **18**(04):1181–211.
32. **Hunt GE, Malhi GS, Cleary M, Lai HMX, Sitharthan T.** Comorbidity of bipolar and substance use disorders in national surveys of general populations, 1990–2015: systematic review and meta-analysis. J Affect Disord. 2016; **206**:321–30.
33. **Berk M, Hallam KT, McGorry PD.** The potential utility of a staging model as a course specifier: a bipolar disorder perspective. J Affect Disord. 2007; **100**(1):279–81.
34. **Cosci F, Fava GA.** Staging of mental disorders: systematic review. Psychother Psychosom. 2012; **82**(1):20–34.
35. **Kapczinski F, Dias VV, Kauer-Sant'Anna M, Frey BN, Grassi-Oliveira R, Colom F,** et al. Clinical implications of a staging model for bipolar disorders. Expert Rev Neurother. 2009; **9**(7):957–66.
36. **Berk M, Berk L, Dodd S, Cotton S, Macneil C, Daglas R,** et al. Stage managing bipolar disorder. Bipolar Disord. 2014; **16**(5):471–7.
37. **Duffy A, Malhi GS, Grof P.** Do the trajectories of bipolar disorder and schizophrenia follow a universal staging model? Can J Psychiatry. 2017; **62**(2):115–22.
38. **Berk M, Conus P, Lucas N, Hallam K, Malhi GS, Dodd S,** et al. Setting the stage: from prodrome to treatment resistance in bipolar disorder. Bipolar Disord. 2007; **9**(7):671–8.
39. **Malhi GS, Byrow Y, Fritz K, Berk L, Berk M.** Does irritability determine mood depending on age? Aust NZ J Psychiatry. 2017; **51**(3):215–6.
40. **Skjelstad DV, Malt UF, Holte A.** Symptoms and signs of the initial prodrome of bipolar disorder: a systematic review. J Affect Disord. 2010; **126**(1):1–13.

41. **Malhi GS, Bargh DM, Coulston CM, Das P, Berk M.** Predicting bipolar disorder on the basis of phenomenology: implications for prevention and early intervention. Bipolar Disord. 2014; **16**(5):455–70.
42. **Correll CU, Hauser M, Penzner JB, Auther AM, Kafantaris V, Saito** E, et al. Type and duration of subsyndromal symptoms in youth with bipolar I disorder prior to their first manic episode. Bipolar Disord. 2014; **16**(5):478–92.
43. **Malhi GS, Bargh DM, Cashman E, Frye MA, Gitlin M.** The clinical management of bipolar disorder complexity using a stratified model. Bipolar Disord. 2012; **14**(s2):66–89.
44. **Berns GS, Nemeroff CB.** The neurobiology of bipolar disorder. Am J Med Genet C Semin Med Genet. 2003; **123C**(1):76–84.
45. **Strakowski SM, DelBello MP, Sax KW, Zimmerman ME, Shear PK, Hawkins JM**, et al. Brain magnetic resonance imaging of structural abnormalities in bipolar disorder. Arch Gen Psychiatry. 1999; **56**(3):254–60.
46. **Hallahan B, Newell J, Soares JC, Brambilla P, Strakowski SM, Fleck DE**, et al. Structural magnetic resonance imaging in bipolar disorder: an international collaborative mega-analysis of individual adult patient data. Biol Psychiatry. 2011; **69**(4):326–35.
47. **Phillips ML, Swartz HA.** A critical appraisal of neuroimaging studies of bipolar disorder: toward a new conceptualization of underlying neural circuitry and a road map for future research. Am J Psychiatry. 2014; **171**(8):829–43.
48. **D'Avanzato C, Joormann J, Siemer M, Gotlib IH.** Emotion regulation in depression and anxiety: examining diagnostic specificity and stability of strategy use. Cognit Ther Res. 2013; **37**(5):968–80.
49. **Ochsner KN, Gross JJ.** The neural architecture of emotion regulation. In: **Gross JJ**, editor. Handbook of emotion regulation. New York, NY: Guilford Press; 2007. p. 87–109.
50. **Pizzagalli DA.** Frontocingulate dysfunction in depression: toward biomarkers of treatment response. Neuropsychopharmacology. 2011; **36**(1):183–206.
51. **Roiser JP, Sahakian BJ.** Hot and cold cognition in depression. CNS Spectrums. 2013; **18**(03):139–49.
52. **Strakowski SM, Adler CM, Almeida J, Altshuler LL, Blumberg HP, Chang KD**, et al. The functional neuroanatomy of bipolar disorder: a consensus model. Bipolar Disord. 2012; **14**(4):313–25.
53. **Malhi GS, Byrow Y, Fritz K, Das P, Baune BT, Porter RJ**, et al. Mood disorders: neurocognitive models. Bipolar Disord. 2015; **17**(S2):3–20.
54. **Hegerl U.** Largely unnoticed flaws in the fundamentals of depression diagnosis: the semantics of core symptoms. Aust NZ J Psychiatry. 2014; **48**(12):1166.
55. **Heller AS, Johnstone T, Peterson MJ, Kolden GG, Kalin NH, Davidson RJ.** Increased prefrontal cortex activity during negative emotion regulation as a predictor of depression symptom severity trajectory over 6 months. JAMA Psychiatry. 2013; **70**(11):1181–9.
56. **Nolen-Hoeksema S.** The role of rumination in depressive disorders and mixed anxiety/depressive symptoms. J Abnorm Psychol. 2000; **109**(3):504.
57. **Joormann J.** Cognitive inhibition and emotion regulation in depression. Curr Dir Psychol Sci. 2010; **19**(3):161–6.

58. **Whitton AE, Treadway MT, Pizzagalli DA.** Reward processing dysfunction in major depression, bipolar disorder and schizophrenia. Curr Opin Psychiatry. 2015; **28**(1):7.
59. **Grotegerd D, Stuhrmann A, Kugel H, Schmidt S, Redlich R, Zwanzger P**, et al. Amygdala excitability to subliminally presented emotional faces distinguishes unipolar and bipolar depression: an fMRI and pattern classification study. Hum Brain Mapp. 2014; **35**(7):2995–3007.
60. **Redlich R, Dohm K, Grotegerd D, Opel N, Zwitserlood P, Heindel W**, et al. Reward processing in unipolar and bipolar depression: a functional MRI study. Neuropsychopharmacology. 2015; **40**(11):2623–31.
61. **McGorry PD, Hickie IB, Yung AR, Pantelis C, Jackson HJ.** Clinical staging of psychiatric disorders: a heuristic framework for choosing earlier, safer and more effective interventions. Aust NZ J Psychiatry. 2006; **40**(8):616–22.
62. **McNamara RK, Nandagopal JJ, Strakowski SM, DelBello MP.** Preventative strategies for early-onset bipolar disorder: towards a clinical staging model. CNS Drugs. 2010; **24**(12):983–96.
63. **Kowatch RA, Fristad M, Birmaher B, Wagner KD, Findling RL, Hellander M**, et al. Treatment guidelines for children and adolescents with bipolar disorder. J Am Acad Child Adolesc Psychiatry. 2005; **44**(3):213–35.
64. **Kowatch RA, Suppes T, Carmody TJ, Bucci JP, Hume JH, Kromelis M**, et al. Effect size of lithium, divalproex sodium, and carbamazepine in children and adolescents with bipolar disorder. J Am Acad Child Adolesc Psychiatry. 2000; **39**(6):713–20.
65. **Findling RL, Frazier TW, Youngstrom EA, McNamara NK, Stansbrey RJ, Gracious BL**, et al. Double-blind, placebo-controlled trial of divalproex monotherapy in the treatment of symptomatic youth at high risk for developing bipolar disorder. J Clin Psychiatry. 2007; **68**(5):781–8.
66. **Soreca I, Frank E, Kupfer DJ.** The phenomenology of bipolar disorder: what drives the high rate of medical burden and determines long-term prognosis? Depress Anxiety. 2009; **26**(1):73–82.
67. **Blakemore SJ, Choudhury S.** Development of the adolescent brain: implications for executive function and social cognition. J Clin Psychiatry. 2006; **47**(3–4):296–312.
68. **Berk M, Brnabic A, Dodd S, Kelin K, Tohen M, Malhi GS**, et al. Does stage of illness impact treatment response in bipolar disorder? Empirical treatment data and their implication for the staging model and early intervention. Bipolar Disord. 2011; **13**(1):87–98.
69. **Malhi GS, Gessler D, Outhred T.** The use of lithium for the treatment of bipolar disorder: recommendations from clinical practice guidelines. J Affect Disord. 2017; **217**:266–80.

Chapter 14

Early intervention in personality disorders

John M. Oldham

Introduction

The fifth edition of the American Psychiatric Association's *Diagnostic and Statistical Manual of Mental Disorders* (*DSM-5*) [1] includes, in the general criteria for a personality disorder (PD), that the 'pattern is stable and of long duration, and its onset can be traced back at least to adolescence or early adulthood'. It also states that 'the traits of a personality disorder that appear in childhood will often not persist unchanged into adult life' and that for 'a personality disorder to be diagnosed in an individual younger than 18 years, the features must have been present for at least 1 year' [1, p. 647]. These stipulations were also included in the two previous editions of the diagnostic manual—*DSM-IV* [2] and *DSM-IV-TR* [3]. One unintended consequence of this requirement seems to have been that, for decades, most clinicians assumed that PDs could not be 'officially' diagnosed in any individual under the age of 18, and it is only recently that there has been a groundswell of research and clinical attention to the PDs in the adolescent period [4].

We now know a great deal about the neurobiological maturational process during pre-adolescence and adolescence, and the crucial roles that heritable risk factors *and* environmental experience play in establishing strong foundations for healthy personality functioning. In particular, the importance of steady, caring attachment figures early in life is now unequivocal—to provide a trustworthy model of adult behaviour, as well as to imbue the growing child with the capacity for eventual goal-directed independence, interpersonal effectiveness, and resilience [5]. In addition, however, the interactive attachment process plays a crucial role by providing a safe 'holding' interpersonal environment for the adolescent, as the developing brain of the adolescent establishes the neuroconnectivity needed to regulate behaviour such as reward-seeking, emotion regulation, impulse control, and cognitive functioning [6].

When things go wrong early in life—such as neglect, invalidation, or frank abuse—disruptions in the attachment process are inevitable. It has been determined that about half of all lifetime cases of psychiatric disorders have their onset by age 14, and two-thirds have their onset by age 24 [7]. In many cases, disruptions in attachment may represent the 'environmental toxin' that activates underlying genetic risk factors, resulting in the emergence of major mental illnesses, including schizophrenia, mood disorders, anxiety disorders, and personality disorders. Fonagy and colleagues have persuasively argued that personality development begins early in life, shaped by the infant's interactions with primary caregivers, and that, unfortunately, high percentages of patients with disabling PDs such as borderline personality disorder (BPD) have experienced childhood trauma and develop insecure attachment [8]. Unless there is timely intervention by a substitute or rescue caregiver, the developing child is at great risk to resort to maladaptive behaviour and to expect the world at large to serve up similar experiences of deprivation, mistrust, exploitation, and negativity. The distorted shape of the personality then starts to become apparent, and it is critical that we consolidate valid and reliable ways to identify these early warning signs of emerging pathology that, without intervention, could herald a lifetime of burden and impaired functioning.

The alternative *DSM-5* model for personality disorders

I was fortunate to be appointed as a member of the *DSM-5* Workgroup on Personality and Personality Disorders, a workgroup given the mandate to explore and develop, if possible, a new dimensional model for diagnosing the PDs. The challenges inherent in this task were many, and the controversies in the process have been described [9–11]. In the end, the workgroup developed a 'hybrid' model that reduced the number of categorical diagnoses from ten to six and introduced a set of pathological personality domains and traits, a dimensional component of the new model that provides great flexibility and scope to portray any individual's pathological trait profile, when present. The American Psychiatric Association chose to designate this model as an 'alternative model' and to include it in Section III of *DSM-5*, the section entitled 'Emerging measures and models'. The familiar categorical *DSM-IV-TR* system to diagnose PDs was retained in Section II of *DSM-5*.

The review of the literature carried out by the workgroup led to a consensus that the two most fundamental components of human personality—normal or abnormal—are a sense of self and the nature of one's interpersonal relationships. The workgroup felt that it would be helpful to 'unpack' each component into two subcomponents. A sense of self is comprised of one's identity and one's capacity for self-direction, and interpersonal relationships can be characterized in terms of one's capacity for empathy and one's capacity for intimacy (mutually rewarding, close, lasting relationships). The workgroup developed a 'level of personality functioning scale', and a narrative description of typical functioning in each of the four areas (identity, self-direction, empathy, and intimacy) is provided for each level of functioning: 0 (little or no impairment), 1 (some impairment), 2 (moderate impairment), 3 (severe impairment), or 4 (extreme impairment). Based on data collected by the workgroup, it was determined that for any PD to be diagnosed, moderate or greater impairment in functioning would be required [12].

Impairment in functioning, then, became the first defining criterion (Criterion A) for the presence of a PD according to the alternative model—moderate or greater impairment in personality functioning in at least two of the four areas of identity, self-direction, empathy, and intimacy. The second criterion (Criterion B) for the presence of a PD, according to the alternative model, was then established as the presence of pathological personality traits. In this way, a dimensional trait landscape was introduced, enabling the diagnostician to portray a highly individualized pathological trait profile of any patient. Five sets of personality trait facets were organized under five trait domains: negative affectivity, detachment, antagonism, disinhibition, and psychoticism.

What does this information have to do with the focus of the global roundtable meeting on prevention and early intervention, held in Hong Kong in December 2016? My response to that question is that the template of the alternative model rests on the recognition that the key ingredients to healthy or pathological personality functioning reside in the quality of one's sense of self and of one's interpersonal relationships—fundamentals of behavioural control that derive from neuroregulatory mechanisms being formed during childhood, adolescence, and early adulthood. One example of the usefulness of the alternative model, I would argue, is its focus on the 'healthiness' (or lack of it) of an adolescent's emerging identity, self-directedness, capacity for empathy, and capacity to form close, mutually gratifying interpersonal relationships.

Borderline personality disorder

The most prevalent PD in clinical populations is BPD—a condition, some would say, that best captures the underlying generic core (perhaps a single underlying risk factor) of all PDs [13, 14]. The prevalence of BPD in the general population (1–2 per cent) [15] exceeds that of schizophrenia. BPD has been shown to be moderately heritable [16, 17], and its emergence conforms to the stress/vulnerability model. Heritable endophenotypes emphasized as risk factors for BPD are impulsive aggression and affective instability [18]. Research advances are clarifying our understanding of the neurobiology and pathophysiology of BPD, summarized in a review by Ruocco and Carcone [6]. Genes are tentatively being identified that may be associated with behavioural aspects of BPD. Stress responses may involve imbalanced interactions between cortisol and neural networks involved in cognitive functioning and emotion regulation in patients with BPD, and there may also be insufficient capacity to activate cortical regions important in cognitive control and the regulation of negative emotions.

Using the alternative model, the *DSM-5* Section III diagnosis of BPD can be made according to the abbreviated criteria. Sharp [19] has proposed five 'myths' about adolescent BPD that are pervasive and persistent, and which need to be corrected when encountered:

1. Psychiatric nomenclature does not allow the diagnosis of PD in adolescence. (Not correct, as just discussed. Also see Chapter 15)
2. Certain features of BPD are normative and not particularly symptomatic of personality disturbance. (Research has debunked the belief that the modal adolescent behaves in stormy 'borderline-like' ways [19].)
3. The symptoms of BPD are better explained by traditional Axis 1 disorders. (Studies demonstrate that although certain symptoms of BPD are shared by other disorders such as bipolar II disorder, BPD is a distinct pathological entity [20].)
4. Adolescents' personalities are still developing and therefore too unstable to warrant a PD diagnosis. (The prevalence of fully-expressed BPD in adolescence is well-established [4, 21]. Also see Chapter 15 by Chanen and colleagues in this volume.)
5. Because PD is long-lasting, treatment-resistant, and unpopular to treat, it would be stigmatizing to label an adolescent with BPD. (Treatment that works can be implemented only if a careful diagnosis is made and the adolescent and the family clearly understand the illness.)

Prevention and early intervention

As mentioned, the early histories of patients who develop BPD commonly include experiences of childhood trauma, abuse, or neglect, potentially disrupting the attachment process and resulting in insecure patterns of attachment [8]. These stressful early-life conditions can heighten the likelihood that many types of psychiatric disorders may begin to appear during adolescence, depending on the type of genetic precursor risk factors in a given individual. A number of research groups have highlighted patterns of parent–child relationships that may signal trouble ahead, such as insecure or disorganized attachment to a caregiver, low trust in the caregiver, and high maternal hostility. Parenting behaviours such as low warmth, exertion of control by guilt, high behavioural control itself, intrusiveness, inconsistency, and harsh punishment can also serve as cautionary alerts. Chanen and McCutcheon [4] emphasized the importance of watching for early signs and symptoms similar to the phenotype of BPD. A number of research groups have suggested that early childhood and adolescent 'markers of vulnerability' include problem behaviour during childhood such as controlling behaviour, hostility, mistrust, aggression, anger, affective instability, and an underdeveloped sense of self [4, 21, 22]. Other diagnoses in childhood, such as attention deficit/hyperactivity disorder or oppositional defiant disorder, may also be early signals of the later development of BPD. At any time throughout childhood and adolescence, the appearance of core diagnostic features of BPD such as identity disturbance, inappropriate anger, paranoid ideation, dissociation, chronic feelings of emptiness, and deliberate self-harm should be of concern.

Although effective methods of prevention of BPD are badly needed, they would rely on valid ways to identify those at high risk before the onset of signs and symptoms, such as, for example, specific genetic abnormalities or other biomarkers [23]. However, it is unlikely, given the complexity and the heterogeneity of BPD, that these will be available soon, if ever. We must then rely on early intervention, and here the challenge shifts to education of families, teachers, and clinicians about early signs and symptoms of BPD (or other PDs) such as those already mentioned, and education about BPD itself. Standardized assessment procedures have been developed to guide clinicians in this assessment process (see Sharp and Fonagy [22]). Once identified, children and adolescents at risk should be enrolled in early intervention programmes, more and more of which are becoming available, though still not nearly enough to meet the need. Chanen and colleagues have advocated for years for early intervention, and they have implemented creative and effective programmes, such as an innovative one called Helping Young People Early (HYPE) [21]. Other types of treatment that have been shown to be effective for adults with BPD, including dialectical behaviour therapy (DBT), mentalization-based therapy (MBT), and cognitive analytic therapy (CAT), are being increasingly studied and utilized as methods of early intervention for adolescents who show signs and symptoms of early-onset BPD.

Summary and conclusions

Great progress has been made in our understanding of the personality disorders, and of BPD in particular. As the picture comes into focus, we see that the PDs are not fundamentally different from other categories of mental illness, contrary to the impression to that effect from pre-*DSM-5* days, when the PDs were marooned on Axis II as if different from conditions like mood disorders, anxiety disorders, substance use disorders, eating disorders, the psychoses, and other psychiatric disorders. We also recognize that, frequently, the PDs have their onset during adolescence, putting them in company with over half of all lifetime psychiatric disorders, which have their onset by the very early age of 14. Now that we've 'cleared the air', it is our imperative to pay close attention to risk factors, psychosocial stressors, and early warning signs of potential future PDs. One way to do this is to consider the nature and quality of early aspects of self-confidence and self-directedness in our younger generation, and to look for evidence of their developing capacity to mentalize—to appreciate and want to understand the point of view of others, and to develop friendships that, at least sometimes, deepen and persist. But as parents and families, isn't this what we already do? Of course it is, but it is not so easy to seriously consider that emotional and behavioural problems might not be just a 'passing phase' but, rather, the early signs of a future personality disorder—which, we're increasingly confident, could be 'headed off at the pass' if we see it, name it, and get help.

References

1. **American Psychiatric Association.** Diagnostic and statistical manual of mental disorders. 5th ed. Arlington, VA: American Psychiatric Association; 2013.
2. **American Psychiatric Association.** Diagnostic and statistical manual of mental disorders. 4th ed. Washington, DC: American Psychiatric Association; 1994.
3. **American Psychiatric Association.** Diagnostic and statistical manual of mental disorders. 4th ed. Text rev. Washington, DC: American Psychiatric Association; 2000.
4. **Chanen AM, McCutcheon LK.** Personality disorder in adolescence: the diagnosis that dare not speak its name. Personal Ment Health. 2008; **2**:35–41.
5. **Sharp C, Kim S.** Recent advances in the developmental aspects of borderline personality disorder. Curr Psychiatry Rep. 2015; **17**:17–21.
6. **Ruocco AC, Carcone D.** A neurobiological model of borderline personality disorder: systematic and integrative review. Harv Rev Psychiatry 2016; **24**:311–29.
7. **Kessler RC, Berglund P, Demler O, Jin R, Merikangas KR, Walters EE.** Lifetime prevalence and age-of-onset distributions of DSM-IV disorders in the National Comorbidity Survey Replication. Arch Gen Psychiatry. 2005; **62**:593–602.
8. **Fonagy P, Bateman AW, Lorenzini N, Campbell C.** Development, attachment, and childhood experiences. In: **Oldham JM, Skodol AE, Bender DS**, editors. The American Psychiatric Publishing textbook of personality disorders. 2nd ed. Washington, DC: American Psychiatric Publishing; 2014.
9. **Silk KR.** Personality disorders in DSM-5: a commentary on the perceived process and outcome of the proposal of the Personality and Personality Disorders Work Group. Harv Rev Psychiatry. 2016; **24**:e15–21.

10. **Skodol AE, Morey LC, Bender S, Oldham JM.** The ironic fate of the personality disorders in *DSM-5*. PDTRT. 2013; **4**:342–9.
11. **Zachar P, Krueger RF. Kendler KS.** Personality disorder in DSM-5: an oral history. Psychol Med. 2016; **46**:1–10.
12. **Morey LC, Bender DS, Skodol AE.** Validating the proposed Diagnostic and Statistical Manual of Mental Disorders, 5th edition, severity indicator for personality disorder. J Nerv Ment Dis. 2013; **201**:729–35.
13. **Reichborn-Kjennerud T, Ystrom E, Neale MC, Aggen SH, Mazzeo SE, Knudsen PG,** et al. Structure of genetic and environmental risk factors for symptoms of DSM-IV borderline personality disorder. JAMA Psychiatry. 2013; **70**:1206–14.
14. **Sharp C, Wright A, Fowler C, Frueh C, Allen J, Oldham JM,** et al. The structure of personality pathology: both general ('g') and specific ('s') factor? J Abnorm Psychol. 2015; **124**:387–98.
15. **Torgersen S.** Prevalence, sociodemographics, and functional impairment. In: **Oldham JM, Skodol AE, Bender DS,** editors. The American Psychiatric Publishing textbook of personality disorders. 2nd ed. Washington DC: American Psychiatric Publishing; 2014.
16. **Amad A, Ramoz N, Thomas P, Jardri R, Gorwood P.** Genetics of borderline personality disorder: systematic review and proposal of an integrative model. Neurosci Biobehav Rev. 2014; **40**:6–19.
17. **Distel MA, Ligthart L, Martin NG, Trull TJ.** Genetc covariance structure of the four main features of borderline personality disorder. J Personal Disord. 2010; **24**:427–44.
18. **Siever LJ, Torgersen S, Gundreson JG, Livesley J, Kendler KS.** The borderline diagnosis III: identifying endophenotypes for genetic studies. Biol Psychiatry. 2002; **51**:964–8.
19. **Sharp C.** Bridging the gap: the assessment and treatment of adolescent personality disorder in routine clinical care. Arch Dis Child. 2017; **102**:103–8.
20. **Paris J, Black DW.** Borderline personality disorder and bipolar disorder: what is the difference and why does it matter? J Nerv Ment Dis. 2015; **203**:3–7.
21. **Chanen A, Berk M, Thompson K.** Integrating early intervention for borderline personality disorder and mood disorders. Harv Rev Psychiatry. 2016; **24**:330–41.
22. **Sharp C, Fonagy P.** Practitioner review. Borderline personality disorder in adolescence: recent conceptualization, intervention, and implications for clinical practice. J Child Psychol Psychiatry. 2015; **56**:1266–88.
23. **Stepp SD, Lazarus SA, Byrd AL.** A systematic review of risk factors prospectively associated with borderline personality disorder: taking stock and moving forward. PDTRT. 2016; **7**:316–23.

Chapter 15

Early detection and timely intervention for borderline personality disorder

Andrew Chanen

Introduction

It is now well established that borderline personality disorder (BPD) is a reliable, valid, and common diagnosis, and a severe and treatable mental disorder [1]. Moreover, evidence suggests that BPD captures a general severity factor that is common to all personality disorders [2]. As such, the terms 'borderline' and 'severe' personality disorder are used interchangeably in this chapter.

Although BPD usually has its onset in the period between puberty and emerging adulthood (i.e. young people) [3], its diagnosis is often delayed and specific treatment is only offered late in the course of the disorder, to relatively few individuals, and often in the form of inaccessible, highly specialized, and expensive services [4]. Convincing evidence indicates that BPD is associated with harms from its earliest stages and that the common practice of 'late intervention' (or no intervention) serves to reinforce functional impairment, disability, and therapeutic pessimism.

Borderline personality disorder is non-normative

BPD is neither a variant of normal adolescent development, nor a 'passing phase' of little consequence. There exists a coherent literature demonstrating that young people with BPD differ from their healthy peers on numerous parameters [5], including impulsivity [6], substance use [7], sexual behaviour [8], rates of self-mutilation and suicide attempts [9, 10], and interpersonal and vocational dysfunction [11].

Recently, it has been recommended that personality disorder research and treatment shifts from a narrow focus on *adolescent* BPD [12], in recognition of studies from sociology, developmental psychology, and developmental neuroscience [13–16] that all point to an extended but coherent period of development from puberty through to around the mid 20s, in economically developed societies. Therefore, more natural developmental periods for research and treatment would be childhood, youth (adolescents and emerging adults), adulthood, and old age.

The personal and societal costs of borderline personality disorder

BPD is associated with severely detrimental personal, social, and economic costs. These include severe and enduring functional disability [17], high burden on families and others [18], physical ill-health [19], greater burden of mental-state disorders, recurrent self-harm, a suicide rate of around 8 per cent [1, 20], and high direct healthcare resource use and costs [21]. Most of the high costs of BPD are actually due to indirect costs, principally work-related disability [e.g. 22]. Individuals with BPD have significant disruption in education, achieve fewer qualifications, and have high levels of unemployment [17, 23, 24]. BPD also shows a strong association with the number of days of lost role functioning [25] and more strongly predicts reliance on disability support than do depressive or anxiety disorders [26].

Notwithstanding these harmful consequences and high costs, the diagnosis and treatment of BPD is usually delayed, and discrimination against people with BPD is endemic. This only serves to deny people with BPD access to effective care at the earliest possible juncture.

Opportunities for prevention and early intervention

Over the past two decades, the explosion of knowledge about personality disorder (especially BPD) in young people [e.g. 27, 28–30] has provided solid ground for early diagnosis and treatment of both subthreshold borderline personality pathology ('indicated prevention') and full-syndrome disorder ('early intervention') [3]. These data have recently been summarized by Chanen and colleagues [31].

There is now unambiguous evidence that personality disorder can be diagnosed in young people. Data show that personality disorder begins in childhood and adolescence, and changes across the life course, with no sudden change in personality development at age 18 years. There is an established normative rise in borderline personality pathology at puberty, peaking in the teenage years and declining thereafter. The prevalence of BPD among adolescents is estimated to be 1–3 per cent in the community, but rises to 11–22 per cent in outpatients and

33–49 per cent in inpatients [3, 27, 28]. Furthermore, *DSM-5* BPD is as valid and reliable a diagnosis in adolescence as it is in adulthood, based on: evidence for its genetic basis; similarity in prevalence, phenomenology, stability, and risk factors; evidence for marked separation of course and outcome of adolescent BPD and other disorders; and efficacy of disorder-specific treatment. Moreover, the 'first wave' of evidence-based treatments has demonstrated that structured treatments for BPD in young people are effective [4]. This has led the *DSM-5* and UK and Australian national treatment guidelines to 'legitimize' the diagnosis of BPD prior to age 18 [32, 33].

BPD is also a legitimate differential diagnosis among the common mental disorders in young people. BPD in young people places a substantial burden on the individual, families, communities, and mental health systems immediately and in the long term. Although BPD is rarely measured in studies of the burden of disease, among 15- to 34-year-old Australians, it is the fourth leading cause of disability-adjusted life years (DALYs) for females and the sixth leading cause for males [34]. Predictably, BPD is associated with very high direct healthcare costs for families and communities [35].

A pragmatic approach to prevention and early intervention

These data suggest that BPD is a prime candidate for prevention and early intervention programmes. Also, BPD is often associated with help-seeking (cf. schizotypal or antisocial PDs [36]), and there is considerable flexibility and malleability of BPD traits in youth [37], making this a key developmental period during which to intervene. Prevention and early intervention for BPD should primarily aim to alter the life-course trajectory of young people with borderline personality pathology by attenuating or averting associated adverse outcomes and promoting more adaptive developmental pathways [3]. It should not be narrowly focused upon the diagnostic and symptomatic features of BPD, as these naturally attenuate over time [29]. Also, it should not be confined to the individual diagnostic 'silo' of BPD. Rather, prevention and early intervention for BPD needs to be integrated into prevention for the full range of mental disorders [38].

The Global Alliance for Prevention and Early Intervention for BPD (GAP) has outlined key clinical, research, social, and policy priorities (see Boxes 15.1–15.3) for prevention and early intervention for BPD, and has provided an agenda to address these [31]. The long-term goal for GAP is to lessen the burden of disease among individuals with BPD, those who care for them, and society at large.

Box 15.1 Global Alliance for Prevention and Early Intervention for BPD: clinical priorities

1. *Early intervention* (i.e. diagnosis of and treatment for BPD when an individual first meets *DSM-5* criteria for the disorder, regardless of their age), as already specified in some national guidelines [32, 33] should be a routine part of clinical practice in child and youth mental health practice.
2. Promising evidence-based interventions have been developed for BPD in young people [50]. *Training of mental health professionals* in these treatment approaches should be prioritized.
3. On the basis of current evidence, *indicated prevention* represents the best starting point towards developing a comprehensive prevention strategy for BPD. Indicated prevention involves preventing the onset of new 'cases' of disorder by targeting individuals showing features of BPD but who do not meet the threshold for a formal diagnosis of BPD (i.e. subthreshold cases).
4. *Failure to encourage appropriate early identification*: the lack of recognition of the validity of BPD and its rightful place among the severe mental disorders affecting youth is problematic. Knowledge about BPD in young people, and its precursor signs and symptoms, should be disseminated among child and youth mental health professionals and among trainees in these professions. Such workforce development strategies should address clinician-centred discomfort with the label, mistaken beliefs, and prejudicial and discriminatory attitudes and behaviour.
5. *Do not delay the diagnosis of BPD*. While this delay in diagnosis might be well-intentioned (e.g. 'protecting' patients from stigma), stigma is an insufficient reason for delay. Non-diagnosis of BPD is discriminatory because it denies individuals the opportunity to make informed and evidence-based treatment decisions, and excludes BPD from healthcare planning, policy, and service implementation. Ultimately, this is harmful to the prospects of these young people.
6. *Misleading terms, or the intentional use of substitute diagnoses, should be discouraged*. Given the evidence for the validity of the BPD diagnosis in this age group, this term should be used. When subthreshold BPD is present, terms such as 'BPD features' or 'borderline pathology' are preferred.
7. *Family and friends should be actively involved* as collaborators in prevention and early intervention for BPD. Typically, family and friends are the 'front line' for young people with BPD, and their central role should be recognized and supported. Modifications to the family environment can be effective in promoting improvement of young people's and family members' mental health.

Adapted from *World Psychiatry*, 16, 2, Chanen AM, Sharp C, Hoffman P., Global Alliance for Prevention and Early Intervention for Borderline Personality Disorder. Prevention and early intervention for borderline personality disorder: a novel public health priority, pp. 215–216.

Box 15.2 Global Alliance for Prevention and Early Intervention for BPD: research priorities

1. *Prevention and early intervention for BPD must be integrated with similar efforts for the other severe mental disorders, such as mood and psychotic disorders.* Integration of these preventative efforts acknowledges the 'equifinal' and 'multifinal' pathways for the development of psychopathology. This is especially important for the future development of universal (whole population) and selective (targeting those with risk factors, but no disorder) prevention, where BPD should be measured as both a predictor and an outcome for prevention programmes.
2. Two approaches can be followed to *building a knowledge base for a healthcare system response to prevention and early intervention for BPD.*
   a. For indicated prevention and early intervention, a critical task is to identify risk factors for the persistence or worsening of problems, rather than the 'onset' or incidence of disorder per se.
   b. Another avenue involves developing interventions based upon causal mechanisms that underlie risk, such as environmental adversities or biomarkers.
3. *Develop and evaluate novel, low-cost preventative interventions that can be widely disseminated.* Such interventions will need to be developmentally appropriate, and stage-/phase-specific, incorporating stepped-care service models. A key principle of this approach is that treatment needs will differ by stage, with more benign and less intensive treatments for early and/or less severe presentations.
4. Programmes offering *education and skills for families* with a young person with BPD are a key priority for treatment research.
5. Research needs to *document the educational, vocational, and social outcomes* for young people with BPD.
6. Further *development and validation of brief and 'user-friendly' assessment tools* is needed to promote the systematic use of standardized assessments in research and clinical settings.
7. *Detailed health economic data are needed* to support prevention and early intervention programmes for BPD. Health economic analyses should be included in all clinical trials.
8. Research is needed to *identify methods to improve access to evidence-based treatments and to reduce dropout from treatments.* This should include novel locations and formats for delivery of treatments, such as in schools, out-of-home care, or youth forensic settings.

Adapted from *World Psychiatry*, 16, 2, Chanen AM, Sharp C, Hoffman P., Global Alliance for Prevention and Early Intervention for Borderline Personality Disorder. Prevention and early intervention for borderline personality disorder: a novel public health priority, pp. 215–216.

Box 15.3 Global Alliance for Prevention and Early Intervention for BPD: social and policy priorities

1. BPD needs to be recognized as a severe mental disorder at all levels of the health system.
2. Evidence-based policy is needed to address BPD from primary through to specialist care, with the aim of building a healthcare system response to prevention and early intervention for BPD, with young people and those who care for them as its focus. Young people and families should be included as partners in the design of such systems.
3. Discriminatory practices in healthcare systems must be eliminated as a priority. Top priority should be given to eliminating BPD being regarded as a 'diagnosis of exclusion' and to the refusal, in some jurisdictions, of health-insurance coverage for people with BPD.

Adapted from *World Psychiatry*, 16, 2, Chanen AM, Sharp C, Hoffman P., Global Alliance for Prevention and Early Intervention for Borderline Personality Disorder. Prevention and early intervention for borderline personality disorder: a novel public health priority, pp. 215–216.

Early detection and intervention in practice

Early detection and intervention for BPD is now justified and realistic in youth (adolescence and emerging adulthood) [31]. Over the past two decades, the Helping Young People Early (HYPE) programme has been developed and researched in Melbourne, Australia [39]. HYPE is a comprehensive and integrated *indicated prevention* and *early intervention* programme for youth (15–25 years of age). This programme should be differentiated from conventional BPD treatment programmes that are applied to individuals who have established, enduring, complex, and severe BPD but who happen to be less than 18 years old. Treatment for this latter group should already be considered part of routine clinical practice in child and youth mental health [3].

HYPE is comprised of a service model and an individual therapy, and incorporates the principles of cognitive analytic therapy (CAT) [40] into both components. CAT is a time-limited, integrative psychotherapy that arose from a theoretical and practical integration of elements of psychoanalytic object relations theory and cognitive psychology, subsequently developing into an integrated model of development and psychopathology [41]. CAT is practical and collaborative in style, with a particular focus upon understanding the individual's problematic interpersonal and self-management relationship patterns and the thoughts, feelings, and behaviours that result from these patterns. A crucial feature of CAT is the joint (patient–therapist) creation of a shared understanding of the patient's problems and their developmental origins, through the use of plain-language written and diagrammatic 'reformulations'. These create the basis for understanding relationship and self-management problems within therapy and in the patient's daily life. They assist the patient to recognize and to revise these dysfunctional relationship patterns. They also assist the therapist to avoid or to recover from collusion with the identified relationship patterns.

CAT has specific advantages in early intervention for BPD, particularly because its integrative and *transdiagnostic* approach can incorporate, within the overall treatment model, the many co-occurring problems (such as mental state disorders, substance use, other personality pathology) that are usual in this patient group. Also, CAT conceives 'psychological mindedness' to be a goal of therapy, not a prerequisite. Youth with BPD seldom present as 'ready' for therapy, and often they have limited and/or adverse experiences of mental health services or therapy. Although CAT is largely a talking-based therapy, it can be modified for use with patients with less verbal capacities and/or for individuals with low IQ or learning difficulties. Finally, CAT is versatile because it is able to encompass many other therapeutic techniques (e.g. cognitive and behavioural) within its overall framework.

Routinely, 16 CAT sessions (plus whatever clinical case management is required) are offered to each patient, with four post-therapy follow-up sessions (at one, two, four, and six months) to monitor progress and risk. This is negotiable to fewer sessions, especially for those who are ambivalent about treatment, but can be extended up to 24 sessions, if needed.

Principles of indicated prevention and early intervention for borderline personality disorder

The treatment literature for BPD overwhelmingly emphasizes provision of individual psychotherapy, leading to the misleading conclusion that lengthy individual therapy is both necessary and sufficient for the treatment of all individuals with BPD. Little weight is given to the model of service delivery that might support the provision of individual therapy for BPD [42], despite the evidence that 'high quality care' for BPD might be as effective as 'branded' psychotherapies [4, 43] or that intermittent care might be effective [4].

The HYPE model of care addresses these issues by defining a model of clinical service delivery that is separate from, but integrated with, provision of individual psychotherapy, through the common language and tools of CAT. HYPE also uses time-limited, intermittent treatment as its primary mode of intervention. Some key features of this model are outlined here.

HYPE adopts a dimensional view of BPD, recognizing the clinical significance of subthreshold features of BPD [44] and also its heterogeneity and 'comorbidity'. This approach combines *indicated prevention* of subsyndromal BPD and *early intervention* syndromal for full-syndrome BPD. One advantage of this is that it avoids unnecessary disputes about eligibility thresholds based on diagnostic criteria when there is a clear need for care.

HYPE aims to 'fit the treatment to the patient' (not vice versa) because the very nature of BPD makes it unrealistic to expect young people with the disorder to possess the self-management capabilities for regular attendance in the early phases of treatment. On the contrary, increased capacity for self-management and care is a goal of treatment. HYPE adopts a flexible (time and location of appointments) and transparent (processes and policies) approach to engagement. When clinicians' needs (e.g. duty of care) might be experienced as being at odds with the patient's expressed needs, this is acknowledged. The CAT model facilitates this discussion through the early establishment of common ground. Similarly, expectations about and tolerance for disruptive behaviour need to match the phase of intervention, while always being mindful of the safety of patients, families, and staff. The early, joint development of a shared understanding of the patient's difficulties is used to promote this discussion and allows the therapist to be aware of collusion with the patient's dysfunctional relationship patterns.

Early intervention programmes need to be offered to everyone presenting for care, rather than 'cherry picking' participants based upon non-evidence-based assumptions or judgemental attitudes about 'suitability' for therapy. Access to and use of high-quality care does not require a commitment to regular psychotherapy. Not everyone who is offered intervention will accept it, and 'easy access' needs to be complemented by a mechanism for 'easy exit' (accompanied by an invitation to return if needed) after a defined period of energetic attempts at engagement. Also, because 'comorbidity' is usual in BPD, there should be limited exclusions based upon psychopathology, such as substance use or antisocial behaviour. These should be addressed within the overall treatment plan, rather than fragmenting the patient's care, which only increases the potential for miscommunication among the multiple agencies that are usually involved. The HYPE clinical case manager/therapist adopts an open, transparent, and collaborative approach with all concerned, using the jointly (patient and clinician) constructed reformulation (with consent) to promote a shared understanding of difficulties, which ensures that all are 'singing from the same song sheet', minimizing professional disputes or 'splits' [45]. This approach also facilitates advocacy on behalf of the young person.

Time-limited intervention is a means of providing the young person with an opportunity to practise what they have learned in treatment, and also serves to limit the potential for iatrogenic harm. It also creates a climate of expectation that the young person will go on to live a fulfilling and functional life, avoiding prolonged and/or collusive relationships with the healthcare system. Practically, it also increases the capacity of the programme to see sufficient numbers of individuals to achieve its prevention aims. The clinical experience at HYPE is that most youth drop in and out of treatment and prefer time-limited therapy contracts. This does not preclude future episodes of CAT, either completing the balance of the 16-session intervention or in the form of 'booster' sessions. The emphasis in CAT is upon having an agreed ending and ending well, which is usually achieved.

A central figure in HYPE's integrated, team-based treatment model is the clinical case manager, who provides both individual psychotherapy and clinical case management. Although they are combined, the model clearly distinguishes between therapy and case management in order to avoid therapy sessions being 'hijacked' by day-to-day crises. All patients are jointly managed with a psychiatrist (or senior psychiatric trainee) and reviewed weekly by the entire treating team. Integrating therapy, case management, and psychiatric care reduces opportunities for professional disputes or 'splits' and helps to reduce direct care costs per patient. It also offers opportunities to generalize progress in therapy to other problems and situations. Finally, and most importantly, a team-based approach offers a supportive environment for clinicians and enables the development of a 'common language' through a shared model of BPD and appropriate interventions for the disorder.

Families are routinely involved in the care of young people in HYPE, informed by the young person's preferences. Although there is a strong focus upon individual sessions, usual practice is to involve families in assessment, treatment planning, and psychoeducation. HYPE routinely offers a multifamily psychoeducation and support group [46]. Where indicated, more formal family intervention sessions are conducted, usually by the primary therapist, using the CAT model. The BPD diagnosis is communicated to patients and families with cautious optimism, based upon the evidence supporting the effectiveness of the HYPE intervention [47, 48].

The HYPE model emphasizes that first-line management for BPD is psychosocial treatment, not medications [49]. Discussion with patients, families, and professionals highlights prescribing hazards, such as polypharmacy, overdose, and misuse. However, medication might be warranted (as an adjunct to psychosocial treatment) for patients who have a co-occurring mental state disorder, such as major depression. Medication use in HYPE involves establishing clear and collaborative goals that are regularly reviewed with the patient. Single drugs are usually prescribed in limited quantities, for a limited time, and ineffective or inappropriate medications are ceased.

Written management plans are developed for all patients (after discussion with and agreement) and are made available electronically to all members of the clinical team. These outline the jointly developed formulation, current management, and specific management recommendations for acute crises, which are based upon the shared formulation and goals. HYPE's primary aim is to foster adaptive self-management for community living and to minimize the risk of iatrogenic harm. Inpatient care is usually only used when all options for community treatment have been exhausted. Admission to hospital is rare and usually voluntary, brief (one to two days), and has specific goals. HYPE clinical case managers work with staff to facilitate a 'common language', to minimize collusion with patients' problems, and to effectively achieve the goals of admission.

Treatment fidelity and completion of the tasks of an episode of care are monitored weekly. In common with most successful BPD treatment models, supervision is an integral part of HYPE. It aims to support clinicians, allow time for reflection, and ensure a high standard of care, taking the form of weekly small-group CAT supervision along with individual clinical case-management supervision every two weeks.

Explicit aims of HYPE are to improve functional outcomes, to develop support networks independent of mental health services, to promote adaptive help-seeking, and to avert unhelpful or maladaptive involvement with the health system. Referrals are often made to external, non-mental health networks and to family medical practitioners for post-discharge support. Patients are also encouraged to practise what they have learned in therapy and to delay seeking further psychotherapy until their six-month follow-up review. This does not preclude further case management or treatment of mental state disorders, as necessary. However, this is infrequently required.

Conclusion

Although BPD usually has its onset in young people, its diagnosis and treatment are often delayed. The past two decades has seen a rapid increase in evidence establishing that BPD can be diagnosed in young people and is both continuous with BPD in adults and more notable for its similarities than for any differences. Accordingly, indicated prevention and early intervention has been developed for BPD, exemplified by the HYPE programme. Such intervention is empirically supported and leads to clinically meaningful improvements for patients. However, this approach requires further development and evaluation over longer periods in order to ensure that there are no significant 'downstream' adverse effects. There is still considerable work entailed in terms of treatment development and innovation, and in overcoming challenges to successful translation of evidence into practice. In order to advance early intervention for BPD, access to evidence-based treatments needs to improve, the variety of available treatments needs to increase, treatments need to be matched to individual development and to the phase and stage of disorder, and workforce development strategies need to update knowledge, culture, and practice in relation to BPD in young people [4].

References

1. **Leichsenring F, Leibing E, Kruse J, New AS, Leweke F.** Borderline personality disorder. Lancet. 2011; **377**(9759):74–84.
2. **Sharp C, Wright AG, Fowler JC, Frueh BC, Allen JG, Oldham J,** et al. The structure of personality pathology: both general ('g') and specific ('s') factors? J Abnorm Psychol. 2015; **124**(2):387–98.
3. **Chanen AM, McCutcheon LK.** Prevention and early intervention for borderline personality disorder: current status and recent evidence. Br J Psychiatry. 2013; **202**(S54):s24–s9.
4. **Chanen AM.** Borderline personality disorder in young people: are we there yet? J Clin Psychol. 2015; **71**(8):778–91.
5. **Cohen P, Crawford TN, Johnson JG, Kasen S.** The Children in the Community Study of developmental course of personality disorder. J Personal Disord. 2005; **19**(5):466–86.
6. **Lawrence KA, Allen JS, Chanen AM.** Impulsivity in borderline personality disorder: reward-based decision-making and its relationship to emotional distress. J Personal Disord. 2010; **24**(6):786–99.
7. **Scalzo F, Hulbert CA, Betts J, Cotton SM, Chanen AM.** Substance use in youth with borderline personality disorder. J Personal Disord. 2018; **32**(5):603–17.
8. **Thompson K, Betts J, Jovev M, Nyathi Y, McDougall E, Chanen AM.** Sexuality and sexual health among female youth with borderline personality disorder pathology. Early Interv Psychiatry. 2017 Oct 27. doi: 10.1111/eip.12510. [Epub ahead of print]
9. **Goodman M, Tomas IA, Temes CM, Fitzmaurice GM, Aguirre BA, Zanarini M.** Suicide attempts and self-injurious behaviours in adolescent and adult patient with bordeline personality disorder. Personal Ment Health. 2017; **11**(3):157–63.
10. **Andrewes HE, Hulbert C, Cotton SM, Betts J, Chanen AM.** Relationships between the frequency and severity of non-suicidal self-injury and suicide attempts in youth with borderline personality disorder. Early Interv Psychiatry. 2017 Jul 18. doi: 10.1111/eip.12461. [Epub ahead of print]
11. **Kramer U, Temes CM, Magni LR, Fitzmaurice GM, Aguirre BA, Goodman M,** et al. Psychosocial functioning in adolescents with and without borderline personlity disorder. Personal Ment Health. 2017; **11**(3):164–70.

12. **Chanen AM, Tackett JL, Thompson K.** Personality pathology and disorder in children and youth. In: **Livesley J, Larstone R,** editors. Handbook of personality disorders: theory, research, and treatment. 2nd ed. New York: Guilford Press; 2018.
13. **Arnett JJ.** Emerging adulthood. A theory of development from the late teens through the twenties. Am Psychol. 2000; **55**(5):469–80.
14. **Nelson EE, Leibenluft E, McClure EB, Pine DS.** The social re-orientation of adolescence: a neuroscience perspective on the process and its relation to psychopathology. Psychol Med. 2005; **35**(2):163–74.
15. **Paus T.** Mapping brain maturation and cognitive development during adolescence. Trends Cogn Sci. 2005; **9**(2):60–8.
16. **Steinberg L.** Cognitive and affective development in adolescence. Trends Cogn Sci. 2005; **9**(2):69–74.
17. **Gunderson JG, Stout RL, McGlashan TH, Shea MT, Morey LC, Grilo CM,** et al. Ten-year course of borderline personality disorder: psychopathology and function from the collaborative longitudinal personality disorders study. Arch Gen Psychiatry. 2011; **68**(8):827–37.
18. **Bailey RC, Grenyer BF.** Burden and support needs of carers of persons with borderline personality disorder: a systematic review. Harv Rev Psychiatry. 2013; **21**(5):248–58.
19. **Quirk SE, Stuart AL, Brennan-Olsen SL, Pasco JA, Berk M, Chanen AM,** et al. Physical health comorbidities in women with personality disorder: data from the Geelong Osteoporosis Study. Eur Psychiatry. 2016; **34**:29–35.
20. **Pompili M, Girardi P, Ruberto A, Tatarelli R.** Suicide in borderline personality disorder: a meta-analysis. Nord J Psychiatry. 2005; **59**(5):319–24.
21. **Horz S, Zanarini MC, Frankenburg FR, Reich DB, Fitzmaurice G.** Ten-year use of mental health services by patients with borderline personality disorder and with other axis II disorders. Psychiatr Serv. 2010; **61**(6):612–16.
22. **van Asselt AD, Dirksen CD, Arntz A, Severens JL.** The cost of borderline personality disorder: societal cost of illness in BPD patients. Eur Psychiatry. 2007; **22**(6):354–61.
23. **Winograd G, Cohen P, Chen H.** Adolescent borderline symptoms in the community: prognosis for functioning over 20 years. J Child Psychol Psychiatry. 2008; **49**(9):933–41.
24. **Sansone RA, Sansone LA.** Employment in borderline personality disorder. Innov Clin Neurosci. 2012; **9**(9):25–9.
25. **Jackson HJ, Burgess PM.** Personality disorders in the community: results from the Australian National Survey of Mental Health and Well-Being Part III: relationships between specific type of personality disorder, Axis 1 mental disorders and physical conditions with disability and health consultations. Soc Psychiatry Psychiatr Epidemiol. 2004; **39**(10):765–76.
26. **Ostby KA, Czajkowski N, Knudsen GP, Ystrom E, Gjerde LC, Kendler KS,** et al. Personality disorders are important risk factors for disability pensioning. Soc Psychiatry Psychiatr Epidemiol. 2014; **49**(12):2003–11.
27. **Sharp C, Fonagy P.** Practitioner review: borderline personality disorder in adolescence—recent conceptualization, intervention, and implications for clinical practice. J Child Psychol Psychiatry. 2015; **56**(12):1266–88.
28. **Kaess M, Brunner R, Chanen A.** Borderline personality disorder in adolescence. Pediatrics. 2014; **134**(4):782–93.

29. **Newton-Howes G, Clark LA, Chanen AM.** Personality disorder across the life course. Lancet. 2015; **385**(9969):727–34.
30. **Winsper C, Lereya ST, Marwaha S, Thompson A, Eyden J, Singh SP.** The aetiological and psychopathological validity of borderline personality disorder in youth: a systematic review and meta-analysis. Clin Psychol Rev. 2016; **44**:13–24.
31. **Chanen AM, Sharp C, Hoffman P, Global Alliance for Prevention and Early Intervention for Borderline Personality Disorder.** Prevention and early intervention for borderline personality disorder: a novel public health priority. World Psychiatry. 2017; **16**(2):215–16.
32. **National Health and Medical Research Council.** Clinical practice guideline for the management of borderline personality disorder. Melbourne: National Health and Medical Research Council; 2012.
33. **National Collaborating Centre for Mental Health.** Borderline personality disorder: treatment and management. London: National Institute for Health and Clinical Excellence; 2009. Report No. CG78. Contract No. 78.
34. **The Public Health Group.** The Victorian burden of disease study. Melbourne: Victorian Government Department of Human Services; 2005.
35. **Goodman M, Patil U, Triebwasser J, Hoffman P, Weinstein ZA, New A.** Parental burden associated with borderline personality disorder in female offspring. J Personal Disord. 2011; **25**(1):59–74.
36. **Tyrer P, Mitchard S, Methuen C, Ranger M.** Treatment rejecting and treatment seeking personality disorders: Type R and Type S. J Personal Disord. 2003; **17**(3):263–8.
37. **Lenzenweger MF, Castro DD.** Predicting change in borderline personality: using neurobehavioral systems indicators within an individual growth curve framework. Dev Psychopathol. 2005; **17**(04):1207–37.
38. **Chanen AM, Berk M, Thompson K.** Integrating early intervention for borderline personality disorder and mood disorders. Harv Rev Psychiatry. 2016; **24**(5):330–41.
39. **Chanen AM, McCutcheon LK, Kerr IB.** HYPE: a cognitive analytic therapy based prevention and early intervention program for borderline personality disorder. In: **Sharp C, Tackett JL**, editors. Handbook of borderline personality disorder in children and adolescents. New York: Springer; 2014.
40. **Ryle A, Kerr IB.** Introducing cognitive analytic therapy. Chichester: John Wiley; 2002.
41. **Kerr IB.** Cognitive analytic therapy. Psychiatry. 2005; **4**(5):28–33.
42. **Mulder RT, Chanen AM.** Effectiveness of cognitive analytic therapy (CAT) for personality disorders. Br J Psychiatry. 2013; **202**:89–90.
43. **Bateman AW, Gunderson J, Mulder R.** Treatment of personality disorder. Lancet. 2015; **385**(9969):735–43.
44. **Thompson K, Jackson HJ, Cavelti M, Betts J, McCutcheon L, Jovev M,** et al. The clinical significance of subthreshold borderline personality disorder features in outpatient youth. J Personal Disord. 2018 Jul 23:1–11. doi: 10.1521/pedi_2018_32_330. [Epub ahead of print].
45. **Kerr IB.** Cognitive-analytic therapy for borderline personality disorder in the context of a community mental health team: individual and organizational psychodynamic implications. Br J Psychother. 1999; **15**(4):425–38.

46. **Pearce J, Jovev M, Hulbert C, McKechnie B, McCutcheon L, Betts J**, et al. Evaluation of a psychoeducational group intervention for family and friends of youth with borderline personality disorder. Borderline Personal Disord Emot Dysregul. 2017; **4**:5.
47. **Chanen AM, Jackson HJ, McCutcheon L, Dudgeon P, Jovev M, Yuen HP**, et al. Early intervention for adolescents with borderline personality disorder using cognitive analytic therapy: a randomised controlled trial. Br J Psychiatry. 2008; **193**(6):477–84.
48. **Chanen AM, Jackson HJ, McCutcheon L, Dudgeon P, Jovev M, Yuen HP**, et al. Early intervention for adolescents with borderline personality disorder: a quasi-experimental comparison with treatment as usual. Aust N Z J Psychiatry. 2009; **43**(5):397–408.
49. **Chanen AM, Thompson KN.** Prescribing and borderline personality disorder. Aust Prescr. 2016; **39**(2):49–53.
50. **Chanen AM, Thompson K.** Preventive strategies for borderline personality disorder in adolescents. Curr Treat Options Psychiatry. 2014; **1**(4):358–68.

Chapter 16

Early intervention in underage drinking

Preliminary results in Brazil

Arthur Guerra de Andrade, Erica Rosanna Siu, Carla Dalbosco, Telma Tiemi Schwindt Diniz Gomes, and Paulina do Carmo Arruda Vieira Duarte

Introduction

Although alcohol has been used worldwide for many centuries, its harmful use leads to important health, social, and economic consequences. In 2012, it accounted for almost 6 per cent of all deaths in the world and for 5 per cent of the global burden of disease (GBD) [1]. The World Health Organization (WHO) set, as a target, a 10 per cent reduction in harmful use of alcohol by 2025, and every country is responsible for developing, monitoring, and evaluating public policies to achieve such this goal [2].

In this context, the implementation of early interventions stands out as an interesting approach to reduce harmful use of alcohol, focusing on early recognition, diagnosis, and treatment throughout the course of alcohol use, before serious consequences occur, especially among young people [3–5].

Whilst most surveys of harmful alcohol use have been conducted in high-income countries, the highest burden of death and disability per litre of alcohol consumed occurs in low-income countries. In developing countries, an increase in alcohol use and its related harm are expected [1, 6–8]. In Brazil—the largest middle-income country in Latin America—alcohol use represents a significant problem. For instance, it has the highest rate of alcohol-attributable deaths among adolescents (15–19 years of age) in the Americas [6], which highlights the need to encourage prevention programmes and intervention initiatives. This chapter provides a brief overview of early intervention in harmful alcohol use in the Brazilian scenario, with specific focus on underage drinking, college students, and screening and brief interventions (SBIs).

Harmful use of alcohol in Brazil

The impact of alcohol use on health is determined by the volume of alcohol consumed and the drinking pattern [1]. The two-year average (2008–2010) of total alcohol consumption for young people in Brazil aged up to and including 15 years was 8.7 litres of pure ethanol per person per year. Even though it is higher than the global average of 6.2 litres, for the same period, it is lower than the previous 9.8-litre Brazilian average [1]. A previous study showed that 10 per cent of drinkers accounted for 50 per cent of total alcohol consumed, and people belonging to the 18–29 years age group consumed 40.3 per cent [9].

The prevalence of heavy episodic drinking (HED) must be pointed out, since it is connected to drinking and driving episodes, and to underage drinking. HED exposes the person to risky situations, such as physical health injuries, unprotected or unconsented sex, unwanted pregnancy, alcoholic overdose, violence, and traffic accidents [10]. In Brazil, in 2010, 18 per cent of the population aged up to and including 15 years had consumed 60 grams or more of pure alcohol at least once in the past 30 days—more than twice the world HED prevalence of 7.5 per cent [1]. In the National Health Survey 2013, HED was reported by 51 per cent of drinkers, 43 per cent of whom reported four or more HED occasions. Awfully, HED drinkers were 70 per cent more likely to report driving after drinking [11].

In Brazil, the HED pattern is more common among young people, and particularly underage drinkers and college students. There are external and personal factors influencing underage drinking. Among external factors are the lack of information and positive adult role models, and ease of access. In the personal context, feeling included and self-confident, signalling power and maturity, proving status and escaping reality are some drivers for young people drinking [4, 5].

According to a recent Pan American Health Organization (PAHO) report, among students aged 13 to 17, over 20 per cent of girls and 28 per cent of boys reported having had an episode of drunkenness in their lifetime [6]. In Brazil, the National Survey of School Health 2015 (PeNSE), conducted with 10,926 students in the same age group, showed similar results: 26.9 per cent for girls and 27.5 per cent for boys [12], meaning that at least one in four students has been exposed to risky situations. Another population analysed by PeNSE was ninth-grade students of elementary school (13–15 years old): 25.1 per cent of girls versus 22.5 per cent of boys reported previous-month alcohol use. This gender convergence on alcohol use is a trend that was earlier reported for adults in several countries [13, 14]. Gender equality and women's empowerment, together, may contribute to an increase in alcohol consumption and its related problems [13, 15].

Among college students, alcohol is the most commonly used substance [16]. In Brazil, the first study on alcohol consumption in this population—the 1st Nationwide Survey on the Use of Alcohol, Tobacco and Other Drugs Among College Students in the 27 Brazilian State Capitals—was conducted by the National Secretariat for Drug Policies (SENAD). In summary, 86.2 per cent of students reported having used alcohol at some point in their lifetime [17]; at least one occasion of HED in the previous month was reported by 25 per cent. It is important to highlight that men consumed more alcohol than women, but the difference was very small [18]. Moreover, students consuming alcohol in combination with energy drinks were more likely to have high-risk traffic behaviours—for example, driving at high speed and driving after a HED occasion—than those consuming only alcohol [19].

Socioeconomic factors also play an important role in drinking patterns and alcohol harm. Interestingly, a study with adolescents living in the five geo-economic regions of Brazil, which have a very distinct gross domestic product (GDP), showed that those having a higher socioeconomic status were more likely to drink more. These findings are exactly opposite to those found for developed countries [20]. On the other hand, in São Paulo metropolitan area, most adult drinkers with alcohol-related disturbances (heavy drinking and alcohol-related disorders) belonged to socially disadvantaged neighbourhoods [21].

Taken together, these data reinforce the importance of encouraging programmes and approaches for prevention and treatment that meet individual needs, taking into account socioeconomic aspects and specific populations, as soon as possible.

Early intervention in the harmful use of alcohol

It remains unclear whether effective interventions for adults are effective when applied to young people. Interventions should be tailored for every target group. For instance, strategies used for elementary school students who, in most part, have never had contact with alcohol, should be different from those applied to college students, who are much more susceptible to experimentation [4].

Setting up the minimum age for buying and consuming alcohol, and increasing taxation, seem to be the most effective measures to prevent alcohol abuse. Increasing taxation and prices reduced the overall consumption [22]. Moreover, it was equally effective for both adults and young people [23].

Although restriction of alcohol advertisements appears to be effective for young people, the results were inconsistent [24]. These so-called 'best buys' (e.g. taxation and restriction of availability and advertisements) may not be sufficient to tackle the harmful use of alcohol. For instance, in the WHO European Region there was a decrease in consumption between 1990 and 2014, but the overall age-standardized rate of alcohol-attributable mortality in 2014 was higher [25]. An interesting approach could be the implementation of screening and brief interventions (SBIs) that help to identify individuals at risk and to prevent and reduce the consequences of alcohol consumption [4].

Brazilian programmes to reduce the harmful use of alcohol among young people

Few initiatives have been scientifically evaluated, and three key issues must be addressed on behaviour-change interventions: Does it work? How well does it work? How does it work? [26]

Very important measures have been carried out by the Brazilian government, such as the implementation of Law 11705 in 2008, that bans the sale of alcoholic beverages on federal highways and establishes zero as the legal blood alcohol concentration limit for driving [27]. The so-called 'Dry Law' was further strengthened in 2012 by Law 12760 [28], which increased the fine and authorized the use of evidence (e.g. videos, testimonials) to prove drunkenness of the driver in a criminal process. The recent approval of the Law 13106 (which prohibits and punishes alcohol sale to under 18-year-olds) was also an important achievement to help reduce the harmful use of alcohol, especially among young people [29]. Capital cities, like Rio de Janeiro, São Paulo, and Porto Alegre, have shown a more pronounced reduction in traffic accidents, probably because of greater police oversight.

The Brazilian government have presented the Strategic Action Plan to Tackle Non-communicable Diseases in Brazil 2011–2022, which includes the target of reducing harmful alcohol consumption from 18 per cent (in 2011) to 12 per cent (in 2022).

School-based alcohol programmes have been associated with reduced frequency of drinking [30]. However, there are some challenges for implementation of prevention programmes in Brazilian schools. The difficulties are generally associated with the lack of teaching materials, lack of funds, and the structure of education [31]. The Ministry of Health decided to invest in a European model of a prevention programme called Unplugged, applying it in public schools across three cities in Brazil (São Paulo, São Bernardo do Campo, and Florianópolis). The target audience of the programme were children aged

11 to 14 years. The Unplugged programme was shown to achieve positive results in eight countries, and to be effective in preventing early onset of alcohol, tobacco, and marijuana use [32]. It consisted of weekly lessons, with life skills and normative contents [33, 34]. Teachers reported difficulties in the implementation of #Tamojunto, such as insufficient time to plan the lessons and lack of school support. Some adaptations could improve the program implementation: involvement of teachers and administrators in training courses on alcohol and other drugs, restructuring the general workload of the teachers, and development of school structure and curricula [33].

Concerning college drinking, few intervention initiatives have been reported in Brazil, and it highlights an important research gap to be fulfilled in the near future. Three cross-sectional studies were conducted in 1996, 2001, and 2009, in the University of São Paulo (USP), in order to identify trends and develop prevention and intervention strategies. A study conducted with 266 students from University of São Paulo State (UNESP) has shown interesting results in this regard [35]. The intervention applied was BASICS (Brief Alcohol Screening and Intervention for College Students) [36], and consisted of a two-meeting intervention, lasting up to 50 minutes each, with a 15-day interval. Follow-up was carried out at 12 and 24 months after the baseline interviews. 'At-risk' drinkers (freshmen) receiving the intervention showed reduced amount and frequency of alcohol use [35].

Screening and brief interventions

Important approaches such as screening and brief interventions (SBIs) must also be considered within the context of early intervention in the harmful use of alcohol. SBIs were developed as a comprehensive and integrated approach that can be flexibly applied in diverse clinical care settings and are indicated for individuals at risk of developing substance use disorders, as well as for those that have been diagnosed [37, 38]. The implementation of such tools in primary healthcare has the potential to help professionals to identify and intervene within the general population [39]. Moreover, SBIs' efficacy on alcohol-related harm reduction has been extensively reported elsewhere [40–42]. A recent study showed a reduction of 85 grams in alcohol consumption per week in hazardous or harmful drinkers after SBI [43]. Another advantage of SBIs is that they are tailored for each individual; and each SBI rarely exceeds five meetings, with sessions lasting only up to 45 minutes. Both the short duration and the low cost, when compared to other types of interventions and intensive treatments, make SBIs an economically viable option that produces benefits for the whole society [37, 44].

In spite of all these advantages, the implementation of alcohol SBIs and their adaptation to regional contexts requires collaborative work among academics, health professionals, and specialists, in order to overcome some barriers [45, 46]. SBIs also require referral to specialist services, when needed [47]. SBI approaches require professionals of both health and social services to be prepared to apply brief screening instruments and to identify people at risk or experiencing substance use [38]. The training of professionals capable of applying SBIs is very simple. Strategies to implement SBIs in primary care have been recently reported in several countries, and it is important to establish an effective workflow in order to fit SBIs in the existing clinical model [5, 48, 49].

Difficulties with the organization and administration of SBI instruments in Brazil have also been referred by health-service managers [50]. A recent Brazilian study pointed out that the main barriers to SBI implementation may be related to a lack of motivation to make investments in changing attitudes [51]. Furthermore, researchers have been working on the development of methods of implementation of SBI and referral to treatment in primary health-care settings in Brazil and Latin America. The main limitations identified were insufficient resources (human, financial, structure), lack of integration and intersectional health-care settings, and little participation by physicians [52].

These studies reinforce the importance of investing in and training health-care professionals working with alcohol misuse and its related harm. Notwithstanding, one of the major challenges for the implementation of public policies in Brazil is its continental dimension. As a strategy to reach its target audience and promote their empowerment and awareness towards this important issue, the Brazilian government funded and established partnerships with the Federal University of São Paulo to develop and implement a distance-learning course. The course, entitled 'System for the detection of abusive use and dependence on psychoactive substances: referral, brief intervention, social reinsertion and follow-up—SUPERA', is in its tenth edition and has reached over 90,000 Brazilian professionals working in health and social-assistance fields [53]. A study conducted after the end of the course showed that the majority of the participants (84 per cent) felt able to perform brief intervention and to develop strategies to reduce substance use [54, 55].

While most of the SBI research was conducted in adult populations and settings, the evidence for its efficacy with young people is not robust [3–5].

Conclusions

The impact of the harmful use of alcohol is a highly relevant topic in distinct aspects: individual, family, social, and economic. The Brazilian scenario is rather worrisome, but advances in public policies have been made in order to reduce alcohol harms. Early interventions should have an important impact on reducing alcohol-related harm, especially for vulnerable populations, such as young people.

There is now robust evidence that SBIs can reduce problems related to alcohol use more quickly, and at a lower cost, than intensive treatments. In Brazil, integration and intersectional health-care settings, as well as training of professionals, could be a starting point. Finally, the reduction of harmful alcohol-related consequences requires the joint effort of civil society, government, and the private sector, with the special engagement of public health and research institutes to consolidate evidence-based strategies and measures.

References

1. **World Health Organization (WHO).** Global status report on alcohol and health 2014. Geneva: WHO; 2014.
2. **World Health Organization (WHO).** Global action plan for the prevention and control of noncommunicable diseases 2013–2020. Geneva: WHO; 2013.
3. **Patton R, Deluca P, Kaner E, Newbury-Birch D, Phillips T, Drummond C.** Alcohol screening and brief intervention for adolescents: the how, what and where of reducing alcohol consumption and related harm among young people. Alcohol Alcohol. 2014; **49**(2):207–12.
4. **Stockings E, Hall WD, Lynskey M, Morley KI, Reavley N, Strang J,** et al. Prevention, early intervention, harm reduction, and treatment of substance use in young people. Lancet Psychiatry. 2016; **3**(3):280–96.
5. **Harding FM, Hingson RW, Klitzner M, Mosher JF, Brown J, Vincent RM,** et al. Underage drinking: a review of trends and prevention strategies. Am J Prev Med. 2016; **51**(4 Suppl 2):S148–57.
6. **Pan American Health Organization (PAHO).** Regional status report on alcohol and health in the Americas. Washington, DC: PAHO; 2015.
7. **Shield KD, Monteiro M, Roerecke M, Smith B, Rehm J.** Alcohol consumption and burden of disease in the Americas in 2012: implications for alcohol policy. Rev Panam Salud Publica. 2015; **38**(6):442–9.
8. **Lewer D, Meier P, Beard E, Boniface S, Kaner E.** Unravelling the alcohol harm paradox: a population-based study of social gradients across very heavy drinking thresholds. BMC Public Health. 2016; **16**:599.
9. **Caetano R, Mills B, Pinsky I, Zaleski M, Laranjeira R.** The distribution of alcohol consumption and the prevention paradox in Brazil. Addiction. 2012; **107**(1):60–8.
10. **Rehm J, Baliunas D, Borges GL, Graham K, Irving H, Kehoe T,** et al. The relation between different dimensions of alcohol consumption and burden of disease: an overview. Addiction. 2010; **105**(5):817–43.
11. **Macinko J, Mullachery P, Silver D, Jimenez G, Libanio Morais Neto O.** Patterns of alcohol consumption and related behaviors in Brazil: evidence from the 2013 National Health Survey (PNS 2013). PloS One. 2015; **10**(7):e0134153.

12. **IBGE.** Pesquisa Nacional de Saúde do Escolar 2015 [National Survey of School Health 2015]. Rio de Janeiro: Instituto Brasileiro de Geografia e Estatística (IBGE—Brazilian Institute of Geography and Statistics); 2016.
13. **Silveira CM, Siu ER, Wang YP, Viana MC, Andrade AG, Andrade LH.** Gender differences in drinking patterns and alcohol-related problems in a community sample in Sao Paulo, Brazil. Clinics. 2012; **67**(3):205–12.
14. **Slade T, Chapman C, Swift W, Keyes KM, Tonks Z, Teesson M.** Birth cohort trends in the global epidemiology of alcohol use and alcohol-related harms in men and women: systematic review and metaregression. BMJ Open. 2016; **6**:e011827.
15. **Holmila M, Raitasalo K.** Gender differences in drinking: why do they still exist? Addiction. 2005; **100**(12):1763–9.
16. **NIAAA.** A call to action: changing the culture of drinking at US colleges. Bethesda, MD: US National Institutes of Health, DHHS; April 2002. (NIH publication no. 02–5010).
17. **Andrade AG, Duarte PCAV, Barroso LP, Nishimura R, Alberghini DG, de Oliveira LG.** Use of alcohol and other drugs among Brazilian college students: effects of gender and age. Braz J Psychiatry. 2012; **34**:294–305.
18. **Andrade AG, Duarte PCAV, de Oliveira LG.** I Levantamento Nacional sobre o Uso de Álcool, Tabaco e Outras Drogas entre Universitários das 27 Capitais Brasileiras [1st Nationwide Survey on the Use of Alcohol, Tobacco and Other Drugs among College Students in the 27 Brazilian State Capitals]. Brasilia: Secretaria Nacional de Políticas sobre Drogas—SENAD [National Secretariat for Drug Policies]; 2010.
19. **Eckschmidt F, de Andrade AG, dos Santos B, de Oliveira LG.** The effects of alcohol mixed with energy drinks (AmED) on traffic behaviors among Brazilian college students: a national survey. Traffic Inj Prev. 2013; **14**(7):671–9.
20. **Sanchez ZM, Locatelli DP, Noto AR, Martins SS.** Binge drinking among Brazilian students: a gradient of association with socioeconomic status in five geo-economic regions. Drug Alcohol Depend. 2013; **127**(1–3):87–93.
21. **Silveira CM, Siu ER, Anthony JC, Saito LP, de Andrade AG, Kutschenko A,** et al. Drinking patterns and alcohol use disorders in Sao Paulo, Brazil: the role of neighborhood social deprivation and socioeconomic status. PloS One. 2014; **9**(10):e108355.
22. **Martineau F, Tyner E, Lorenc T, Petticrew M, Lock K.** Population-level interventions to reduce alcohol-related harm: an overview of systematic reviews. Prevent Med. 2013; **57**(4):278–96.
23. **Elder RW, Lawrence B, Ferguson A, Naimi TS, Brewer RD, Chattopadhyay SK,** et al. The effectiveness of tax policy interventions for reducing excessive alcohol consumption and related harms. Am J Prevent Med. 2010; **38**(2):217–29.
24. **Siegfried N, Pienaar DC, Ataguba JE, Volmink J, Kredo T, Jere M,** et al. Restricting or banning alcohol advertising to reduce alcohol consumption in adults and adolescents. Cochrane Database Syst Rev. 2014; (11):Cd010704.
25. **Regional Office for Europe of the World Health Organization (WHO/Europe).** Public health successes and missed opportunities—trends in alcohol consumption and attributable mortality in the WHO European Region, 1990–2014. Copenhagen, Denmark: WHO/Europe; 2016.

26. **Michie S, Abraham C.** Interventions to change health behaviours: evidence-based or evidence-inspired? Psychol Health. 2004; **19**(1):29–49.
27. Brazil. Lei 11.705, de 19 de Junho de 2008 [Law 11705, edited on 19 June 2008]. Diário Oficial da União [Federal Official Gazette of Brazil]; 2008.
28. Brazil. Lei 12.760, de 20 de dezembro de 2012 [Law 12760, edited on 20 December 2012]. Diário Oficial da União [Federal Official Gazette of Brazil]; 2012.
29. Brazil. Lei 13.106, de 17 de março de 2015 [Law 13106, edited on 17 March 2015]. Diário Oficial da União [Federal Official Gazette of Brazil]; 2015.
30. **Das JK, Salam RA, Arshad A, Finkelstein Y, Bhutta ZA.** Interventions for adolescent substance abuse: an overview of systematic reviews. J Adolesc Health. 2016; **59**(4S):S61–75.
31. **Pereira AP, Paes AT, Sanchez ZM.** Factors associated with the implementation of programs for drug abuse prevention in schools. Rev Saude Publica. 2016; **50**:44.
32. **Vigna-Taglianti FD, Galanti MR, Burkhart G, Caria MP, Vadrucci S, Faggiano F**, et al. 'Unplugged', a European school-based program for substance use prevention among adolescents: overview of results from the EU-Dap trial. New Dir Youth Dev. 2014; **2014**(141):67–82, 11–2.
33. **Medeiros PF, Cruz JI, Schneider DR, Sanudo A, Sanchez ZM.** Process evaluation of the implementation of the Unplugged Program for drug use prevention in Brazilian schools. Subst Abuse Treat Prev Policy. 2016; **11**:2.
34. **Kreeft PVD, Wiborg G, Galanti MR, Siliquini R, Bohrn K, Scatigna M**, et al. 'Unplugged': a new European school programme against substance abuse. Drugs. 2009; **16**(2):167–81.
35. **Simao MO, Kerr-Correa F, Smaira SI, Trinca LA, Floripes TM, Dalben I**, et al. Prevention of 'risky' drinking among students at a Brazilian university. Alcohol Alcohol. 2008; **43**(4):470–6.
36. **Dimeff LA, Baer JS, Kivlahan DR, Marlatt GA.** Brief Alcohol Screening and Intervention for College Students (BASICS): a Harm reduction approach. New York: Guilford Press; 1999.
37. **Babor TF, McRee BG, Kassebaum PA, Grimaldi PL, Ahmed K, Bray J.** Screening, Brief Intervention, and Referral to Treatment (SBIRT): toward a public health approach to the management of substance abuse. Subst Abuse. 2007; **28**(3):7–30.
38. **Rush B.** Evaluating the complex: alternative models and measures for evaluating collaboration among substance use services with mental health, primary care and other services and sectors. Nord Stud Alcohol Dr. 2014; **31**(1):27–44.
39. **Cruvinel E, Richter KP, Bastos RR, Ronzani TM.** Screening and brief intervention for alcohol and other drug use in primary care: associations between organizational climate and practice. Addict Sci Clin Pract. 2013; **8**:4.
40. **Alvarez-Bueno C, Rodriguez-Martin B, Garcia-Ortiz L, Gomez-Marcos MA, Martinez-Vizcaino V.** Effectiveness of brief interventions in primary health care settings to decrease alcohol consumption by adult non-dependent drinkers: a systematic review of systematic reviews. Prev Med. 2015; **76** (Suppl):S33–8.
41. **Bertholet N, Daeppen JB, Wietlisbach V, Fleming M, Burnand B.** Reduction of alcohol consumption by brief alcohol intervention in primary care: systematic review and meta-analysis. Arch Intern Med. 2005; **165**(9):986–95.

42. **Kaner EF, Beyer F, Dickinson HO, Pienaar E, Campbell F, Schlesinger C**, et al. Effectiveness of brief alcohol interventions in primary care populations. Cochrane Database Syst Rev. 2007; **2007**(2):CD004148.
43. **McQueen JM, Howe TE, Ballinger C, Godwin J.** Effectiveness of alcohol brief intervention in a general hospital: a randomized controlled trial. J Stud Alcohol Drugs. 2015; **76**(6):838–44.
44. **Babor TF, Higgins-Biddle JC, Dauser D, Burleson JA, Zarkin GA, Bray J.** Brief interventions for at-risk drinking: patient outcomes and cost-effectiveness in managed care organizations. Alcohol Alcohol. 2006; **41**(6):624–31.
45. **Abidi L, Oenema A, Nilsen P, Anderson P, van de Mheen D.** Strategies to overcome barriers to implementation of alcohol screening and brief intervention in general practice: a Delphi study among healthcare professionals and addiction prevention experts. Prev Sci. 2016; **17**(6):689–99.
46. **Kaner E.** NICE work if you can get it: development of national guidance incorporating screening and brief intervention to prevent hazardous and harmful drinking in England. Drug Alcohol Rev. 2010; **29**(6):589–95.
47. **Ronzani TM, Furtado EF.** Estigma social sobre o uso de álcool [Social stigma about alcohol use]. J Bras Psiquiatr. 2010; **59**:326–32.
48. **Kaiser DJ, Karuntzos G.** An examination of the workflow processes of the Screening, Brief Intervention, and Referral to Treatment (SBIRT) Program in health care settings. J Subst Abuse Treat. 2016; **60**:21–6.
49. **Rahm AK, Boggs JM, Martin C, Price DW, Beck A, Backer TE**, et al. Facilitators and barriers to implementing Screening, Brief Intervention, and Referral to Treatment (SBIRT) in primary care in integrated health care settings. Subst Abuse. 2015; **36**(3):281–8.
50. **Ronzani TM, Ribeiro MS, Amaral MB, Formigoni ML.** Hazardous alcohol use: screening and brief intervention as routine practice in primary care. Cad Saude Publica. 2005; **21**(3):852–61.
51. **Amaral MB, Ronzani TM, Souza-Formigoni ML.** Process evaluation of the implementation of a screening and brief intervention program for alcohol risk in primary health care: an experience in Brazil. Drug Alcohol Rev. 2010; **29**(2):162–8.
52. **Antunes da Costa PH, Belchior Mota DC, Cruvinel E, Santana de Paiva F, Ronzani TM.** Developing a method of implementation of screening, brief intervention, and referral to treatment in primary health care settings of Brazil and Latin America. Addict Sci Clin Pract. 2013; **8**(1):A6.
53. **SENAD.** SUPERA: sistema para detecção do uso abusivo e dependência de substâncias psicoativas: encaminhamento, intervenção breve, reinserção social e acompanhamento—9a. edição [SUPERA: system for the detection of abusive use of and dependence on psychoactive substances: referral, brief intervention, social reinsertion and follow-up—9th edition]. 9th ed. Brasilia: Secretaria Nacional de Políticas sobre Drogas—SENAD [National Secretariat for Drug Policies]; 2016.
54. **Souza-Formigoni MLO, Carneiro APL, Silva EA, Duarte PCAV.** Implementation of screening tools and brief intervention by health professionals trained by a distance learning course. Addict Sci Clin Pract. 2012; 7(Suppl 1):A86.

55. **Carneiro APL.** Avaliação da efetividade de um programa de treinamento por educação à distância para capacitação de profissionais de saúde na triagem do uso de álcool e/ou outras drogas e na realização de intervenção breve [Evaluation of the effectiveness of a distance learning program in the training of health professionals in the screening and brief intervention for alcohol and/or other drugs users] [PhD Thesis]. Brazil: Federal University of Sao Paulo; 2014.

Chapter 17

Where next for early intervention programmes?

Dinesh Bhugra, Antonio Ventriglio, and Eric Y.H. Chen

Over the past half century, psychiatry has shifted dramatically, with better knowledge and understanding both of the brain, and its structures and functioning, and of the delivery of services. In the many countries, with the advent of antipsychotic drugs, large institutions which had existed previously to contain people with mental illness started closing, with services moving to general hospitals and community mental-health centres. This was followed by a shift to home treatment and crisis-resolution teams; but over the past two decades, there has been a clear and marked shift to individualized treatment. There has also been a move towards public mental health looking at prevention and early interventions. Early intervention often has been confused with preventative strategies and medication, but as the contributions in this volume show, this is evidently not the case.

This volume has covered many major psychiatric disorders, but not exhaustively, as many other conditions either do not have an evidence base or have not been studied at length. The evidence for early interventions in psychoses probably remains the strongest. There is no doubt that mental illness of varying kinds can contribute to a very heavy burden, both globally and also on individual families and carers who are looking after patients in their prodrome or after they have developed the illness. In many low- and middle-income countries, knowledge about mental illness may be based on religious, natural, and supernatural causation, and may well also rely on an external locus of control which will affect the pathway into care and also therapeutic alliance and adherence.

Role of cultures

Cultures inevitably mould the models of ill health and care, and go on to play a major role in shaping people's expectations of the healthcare and interventions they will receive. Cultures influence individuals' social and cognitive development and, therefore, proceed to affect their 'world view'. Cultures enable individuals to express their distress through various idioms which may be misunderstood in other cultures or may not be understood by those providing healthcare. These idioms can be supernatural, natural, medical, psychological, social, or a mix of these. In addition, they will be coloured by the type of culture—whether it is traditional or modern. These idioms do not map on to traditional classificatory or diagnostic systems, and they influence, very strongly, the pathways patients follow in seeking help and the sources of available help. In addition to moulding the symptoms, cultures also influence the causation, precipitation, and perpetuation of psychiatric symptoms. Social influences on psychiatric symptoms are affected by what cultures define as normal, abnormal, or deviant. These factors will therefore impact upon how diseases are identified.

As described in this volume, there needs to be a distinction made between disease and illness. Clinicians are trained in identifying disease and their focus, by and large, is on pathology, whereas the social impact of disease turns that experience into illness experience, where patients are more interested in getting their social functioning better. Therefore, newer models of early intervention are required which take recovery and improvement in social functioning into account and make these their focus for intervention.

In many parts of the world, minority communities, and especially migrant communities, show higher rates of psychiatric disorders. The models for early intervention for these groups may require a different approach. Pathways into care for minority ethnic groups are different, and these people may enter the formal healthcare system through crisis, justice, or legal systems, and in a compulsory manner. The introduction of early intervention services with their focus on earlier, more collaborative, care might be one model which requires attention, assessment, and evaluation.

Duration of untreated illness

For psychoses, the untreated duration of mental illness can last for years, depending upon the resources available and the models of illness perceived by the patients and their families and carers. The preclinical state is often seen as a non-state and offers a critical threshold. According to resources, cultures will often dictate, in subtle ways, what the threshold is, in order to develop psychiatric services. In many cultures, depending upon the services and personality of individuals, as well as family support, a risk assessment may well contribute to further stress and distress. It may also affect the likelihood of getting health or other insurance, and may lead to personal difficulties such as getting married. Clinicians need to remember that cultural differences in communication between doctors and patients may well contribute to tensions and poor therapeutic engagement if the patients' or their carers' views and explanatory models are not taken into account.

The prodromal phase in psychoses may be prolonged, lasting perhaps for years. The duration of untreated psychoses can also play a role in a decline in social functioning, even though the prodromal phase offers an opportunity for the early detection of psychosis and, thus, indicated prevention. The ultra-high risk (UHR) criteria and basic symptom criteria described in this volume can enable clinicians to identify appropriate individuals for intervention. As the UHR criteria were explicitly developed to predict a first-episode psychosis within 12 months, the attenuated psychotic symptoms (APS) include those which may be similar to positive symptoms such as delusions, hallucinations, and formal thought disorders. Some insight into the illness may be retained. On the other hand, basic symptom criteria aim to detect the increased risk of psychoses at the earliest possible opportunity, with identification of the first subtle disturbances in information processing, which are experienced with full insight. The best option, as noted earlier in this volume, is to recognize these changes before any functional decline and before the individual's coping strategies are totally lost. It is possible that, for vulnerable populations, a combination of both approaches will be most suitable. It is essential that the clinicians are trained to be sensitive to these approaches in the case of vulnerable children and young people.

Bearing in mind that resources for managing mental health are limited globally, working 'outside the box' may be one option. In some low- and middle-income countries, the training of volunteers, school children and teachers, neighbours, religious leaders, and the community at large has proved to be a very useful intervention. More than that, such approaches help to reduce stigma and provide training for early identification, as well as offer individuals a degree of ownership of their own and others' mental health.

Role of stigma

Cultures and societal attitudes to mental illness are affected by stigma and that, in turn, will influence how healthcare systems are developed and how people seek help. The actual presentation and patterns of help-seeking are strongly influenced by local resources. There is no doubt that stigma and discrimination against people with mental illness deters patients, as well as their families, from seeking help. Rarely, in some cultures, those with mental illness are seen in a positive manner (e.g. as having special healing powers or as deities), which may also deter them and their families from seeking help and prevent early interventions from working. However, this is changing, and traditional attitudes are being challenged, as a result of rapid globalization and the increased pace of industrialization and urbanization. Another factor that needs serious consideration is the impact of social media and possible uses of e-mental health, including telemental health.

More often than not, stigma against mental illness can lead to discrimination in all fields of life including marriage, inheriting property, voting, and employment. Unfortunately, stigma can also influence members of patients' families, institutions in which they receive treatment, medications which are used to treat them, and also the health workers who provide care for them. Widespread discrimination and stigma affect research funding and resources for clinical services. Stigmatization is a result of concept formation during which individuals learn to recognize the many and different essential characteristics of a group of individuals or things. Once embedded in the legal system, these attitudes carry very strong values.

In many countries, the long duration of untreated psychosis (DUP) and probable severe consequences have often been at the heart of setting up services which have frequently included comprehensive, integrated, patient-centred programmes, with the aim of improving the outcome of patients with first-episode psychosis through public awareness and destigmatization initiatives. Other countries have had stand-alone services; whereas in many settings, collaboration with community services, and provision of early engagement and phase-specific care of those with psychosis, have been critical. Various models exist: consultation liaison to home treatment and crisis-resolution teams; strategies for early intervention; and more broad-based services with a clear focus on promoting awareness of youth mental health issues and encouraging youth to seek help early, as well as on early intervention and possible prevention strategies.

In many countries both in low- and middle-income settings, as well as in some high-income countries, psychiatric services still remain largely asylum-based. Although attempts are being made to deinstutionalize patients, early interventions have some way to go. The reluctance to seek help, by the patients and their families and carers, contributes to delayed community interventions. It is possible that a lack of literacy about mental illness can contribute to a long DUP. In many countries, the concept of the prodromal state might not yet be widely recognized even among psychiatrists. Closer integration with primary care, better education at undergraduate and postgraduate level, and continuing medical education activities are urgently required in relation to treating and diagnosing mild and moderate disorders, and to building the community-based networks for early detection and early interventions.

Among psychoses, schizophrenia is a complex disorder in which risk genes involved in neuroplasticity are interacting with environmental risk factors and social factors. It is well recognized that schizophrenia and related psychoses are not degenerative in origin, but are disturbances of regenerative/plastic processes of the brain involving neurogenetic events in the dentate region focusing on oligodendrocyte and synaptogenesis-related processes. As discussed in this volume, in order to prevent psychosis, persons at risk need to be identified during the early phases of their illness in order to initiate a phase-specific treatment. Therefore, understanding the mechanisms underlying the development of psychosis and strengthening the plasticity of the brain could effectively stop the progression of psychosis.

Early interventions

On the other hand, the concept of early intervention is also attractive and logical for bipolar disorder (BD). Recognition of symptoms of the onset and resulting delays in seeking help are significant factors. There are many problems in reaching diagnosis early because patients and clinicians alike may see the mood changes without attributing any clinical significance to them. Of course, there is always a theoretical risk in implementing strategies without being clear about what is needed, and how and when early intervention is to be delivered. These risks also include unnecessarily prescribing potentially harmful medication to perhaps inadvertently accelerating the progression of the illness. It is important to recognize that the main goals of early intervention in psychosis (EIP) are to reduce the time period between the onset of psychosis and the commencement of effective treatment, as well as to provide consistent and comprehensive care during the critical early years of illness. The term 'duration of untreated bipolar' (DUB) has been employed, and factors which contribute to conversion of prodromal BD to a syndrome need further research and investigation in young persons in the peak age range for the onset of severe mental disorders.

Alcohol dependence

There is no doubt that alcohol use represents a significant burden. For early interventions in the use of alcohol dependence, an appropriate approach is to reduce harmful use of alcohol by focusing on the early recognition, diagnosis, and treatment across the full trajectory of alcohol use before more severe consequences occur. Early education and a focus on young people (underage and college students) should be given primacy, with a particular emphasis on girls. There is clear and robust evidence that screening and brief interventions can, in quite a short period, help reduce problems related to alcohol use, and at a lower cost, than more intensive treatments later on. Throughout the world, there remain major barriers in implementation of early intervention, especially in primary care services. There is no doubt that alcohol is not only a health issue but also requires civil society, non-governmental organizations, community leaders, and policymakers, with special engagement of public health and research institutes, to consolidate and share evidence-based strategies and measures.

Families have a major role to play in early identification and early engagement with services, and service providers have an obligation to ensure that services are 'fit for purpose'. Families may be supportive, critical, or neutral, but still carry major importance in people's lives. They are often underutilized, even when they are willing to be active partners in managing patients.

Recommendations

If the future of early interventions is to be secure, then we urge the following recommendations.

Researchers

1. More research is needed to explore, in greater depth, the role of various factors in early identification, development, and full emergence of a psychiatric disorder.
2. The funding for research in psychiatric disorders lags woefully behind that of physical illnesses, in spite of the fact that the global burden of disease due to psychiatric disorders is probably highest.
3. Pathways into care in the context of cultural impact on idioms of distress and help-seeking deserve fuller studies as a matter of urgency, so that evidence can guide the service development and provision.
4. The impact of cultural factors on various psychiatric disorders deserves better study.

Clinicians

1. Wherever possible, services should move away from institutionalization to community-based services which can be evaluated, and to the development of specific services such as home treatment and early intervention.
2. Services need equitable funding in order to work with communities to form partnerships with non-governmental organizations, patient and family organiszations, policymakers, employers, and judicial and legal systems.

3. Wherever possible, public education on mental disorders should start at an early age, in schools and parenting classes.
4. Public mental health needs to be integrated with healthcare delivery.
5. Better integration between primary and secondary care is needed.
6. Better integration between psychiatric care and social services, wherever possible, should be encouraged.

Policymakers

1. Policymakers need to help institutions to close, with a move to community care, supported by appropriate and adequate funding and resources.
2. They should take the lead on developing partnerships with key stakeholders.
3. Policymakers must ensure that sufficient funds are available to both mental-health services and also to early-intervention services.
4. Policymakers must include mental health as a priority across all policies.
5. Policymakers can take the lead in developing and delivering on the integration agenda.

Index